Headache

Series Editor:

Paolo Martelletti
Roma, Italy

The purpose of this Series, endorsed by the European Headache Federation (EHF), is to describe in detail all aspects of headache disorders that are of importance in primary care and the hospital setting, including pathophysiology, diagnosis, management, comorbidities, and issues in particular patient groups. A key feature of the Series is its multidisciplinary approach, and it will have wide appeal to internists, rheumatologists, neurologists, pain doctors, general practitioners, primary care givers, and pediatricians. Readers will find that the Series assists not only in understanding, recognizing, and treating the primary headache disorders, but also in identifying the potentially dangerous underlying causes of secondary headache disorders and avoiding mismanagement and overuse of medications for acute headache, which are major risk factors for disease aggravation. Each volume is designed to meet the needs of both more experienced professionals and medical students, residents, and trainees.

More information about this series at http://www.springer.com/series/11801

Antoinette Maassen van den Brink
E. Anne MacGregor

Editors

Gender and Migraine

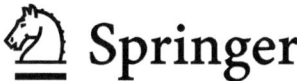 Springer

Editors
Antoinette Maassen van den Brink
Division of Pharmacology
and Vascular Medicine
Erasmus University Medical Center Rotterdam
Rotterdam
The Netherlands

E. Anne MacGregor
Barts Health NHS Trust
London
UK

ISSN 2197-652X   ISSN 2197-6538   (electronic)
Headache
ISBN 978-3-030-02987-6   ISBN 978-3-030-02988-3   (eBook)
https://doi.org/10.1007/978-3-030-02988-3

Library of Congress Control Number: 2019930349

This Springer imprint is published by the registered company Springer Nature Switzerland AG
The registered company address is: Gewerbestrasse 11, 6330 Cham, Switzerland

Foreword

In the last 50 years, medicine has considered and studied patients regardless of gender, sociocultural, and environmental characteristics. Clinical trials are a typical example; experimental clinical studies composed mainly, especially in the phase II studies, voluntary samples of the male population. In migraine, this is not epidemiologically possible, but this reverses and comforts this disparity. The consequence is a reduced personalization and standardization of care measured on the male subject without taking into account variables such as gender, social status, education, culture, education, access to care, and the type of multiple therapies required for intercurrent comorbidity or transient diseases.

This so-called neutral approach of contemporary medicine is badly combined with a disease, migraine, which intersects the patient's entire health life, whatever gender it belongs to or wishes to belong to.

We must therefore speak about gender-specific headache medicine, and this brilliant volume, edited by Antoinette Maassen van den Brink and Anne MacGregor, authoritative area scientists, will help experts to reshape clinical and research activity in the light of this not beyond derogable vision of primary headaches.

Rome, Italy   Paolo Martelletti

Preface

We are delighted to produce this book, dedicated to gender and migraine, endorsed by the European Headache Federation. Migraine is recognized to affect more women than men and is widely considered to be consequent to the effect of female sex hormones. Yet, despite this recognition, basic research still often uses male animal models, without a justification of the sex used. Further, clinical trials fail to analyze data from men and women separately. With increasing numbers of transgender men and women undergoing hormone therapy, we also need to consider how treatment will affect migraine. Moreover, a proper study of the effect of hormone treatment in such specific groups may shed more light on the mechanisms involved in the effects of sex hormones on the pathophysiology of migraine. In this book, we aim to address many of these issues and discuss opportunities for future research.

We are extremely grateful to each of the renowned authors involved in this project who are all experts in their fields. The authors present their personal opinions supported by evidence. Given the variations in drugs and doses worldwide, we urge readers to refer to their local formularies when considering the recommendations presented.

We also thank Angela Schulze-Thomin and Donatella Rizza at Springer, with particular thanks to the project coordinator, Madona Samuel.

Rotterdam, The Netherlands   Antoinette Maassen van den Brink
London, UK   E. Anne MacGregor

Contents

Chapter 1
Epidemiology of Migraine in Men and Women

Kjersti Grøtta Vetvik

1.1 Introduction

Migraine is a primary headache disorder—a headache without underlying cause [1]. The diagnosis is based on the patients' reported symptoms during attacks and can to date not be confirmed by any specific diagnostic tests, e.g., blood tests or radiological investigations.

The International Classification of Headache Disorders (ICHD) defines two major subtypes of migraine which may coexist; migraine without aura and migraine with aura [1]. The main feature of migraine without aura is a unilateral throbbing headache of moderate to severe intensity. Headache is often aggravated by routine physical activity and is accompanied by photo- and phonophobia, as well as nausea with or without vomiting. The migraine headache is thought to be a result of activation of trigeminovascular pathways, the brain stem, and diencephalic nuclei with subsequent release of neuropeptides and sensitization of second- and third-order central neurons [2].

Migraine with aura affects about one third of migraineurs and is characterized by one or more transient and fully reversible focal neurological symptoms developing gradually over minutes, of which each symptom lasts for up to an hour [1, 3, 4]. The most common aura symptoms are visual disturbances, followed by sensory symptoms and speech problems. In rare cases, the migraine aura can also include motor symptoms and retinal or brain stem symptoms. The migraine aura is in most cases followed, by or accompanied by, a headache that may or may not have migrainous features, but in fewer than 5%, no headache occurs [5]. A slowly propagating wave of neuronal depolarization, the so-called

K. G. Vetvik (✉)
Department of Neurology, Akershus University Hospital, Lørenskog, Norway
e-mail: Kjersti.grotta.vetvik2@ahus.no

© Springer Nature Switzerland AG 2019
A. Maassen van den Brink, E. A. MacGregor (eds.), *Gender and Migraine*,
Headache, https://doi.org/10.1007/978-3-030-02988-3_1

cortical spreading depression, is the anticipated underlying pathophysiological mechanism for the aura [6].

Migraine may also be subdivided into episodic and chronic migraine, depending on the total headache frequency per month. Chronic migraine is defined as headache occurring on 15 or more days per month for more than 3 months, which has the features of migraine headache on at least 8 days per month [1]. In episodic migraine, headache occurs less than 15 days per month.

The distinction between episodic and chronic migraine has mainly implications for the treatment, while the subclassification of migraine with and without aura additionally is relevant to comorbidity, assessment of risk factors (e.g., vascular diseases), and prognosis—especially in women.

1.2 Prevalence of Migraine

The prevalence of migraine is significantly influenced by age and sex. In prepubertal children, the prevalence is about 3–7% with no significant difference between boys and girls [7–11]. From the age of 10–14 years, and during all the following years, the prevalence is two to three times higher in women than in men. The maximum sex difference is between age 30 and 45 (Fig. 1.1) when the migraine prevalence peaks in both men and women [12–16]. After the age of 50 years, the prevalence declines in both sexes, most markedly for women. New onset of migraine after the age of 50 years is rare in both sexes [17].

The prevalence of migraine varies across continents with the highest figures in Australia, Europe, and North America and the lowest in Africa, Central/South America, and Southeast Asia (Fig. 1.2a, b). The male to female prevalence ratio is

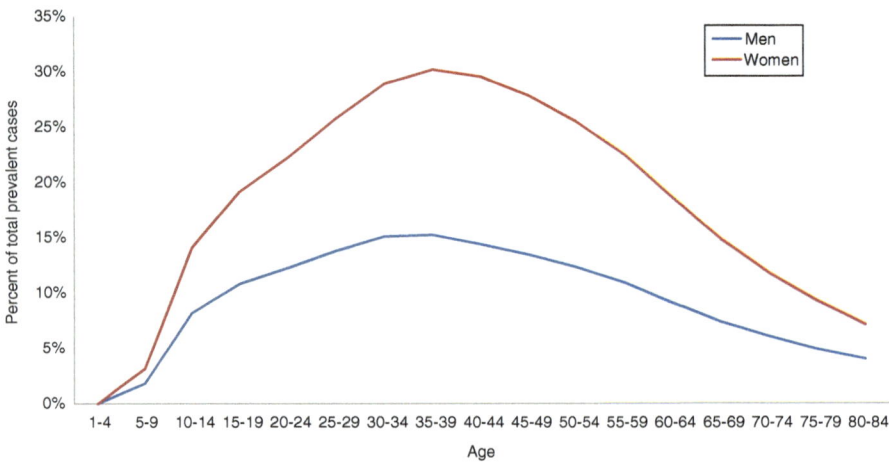

Fig. 1.1 Prevalence of migraine by age and sex. Data from the Global Burden of Disease Study 2016 (GBD 2016) [18]

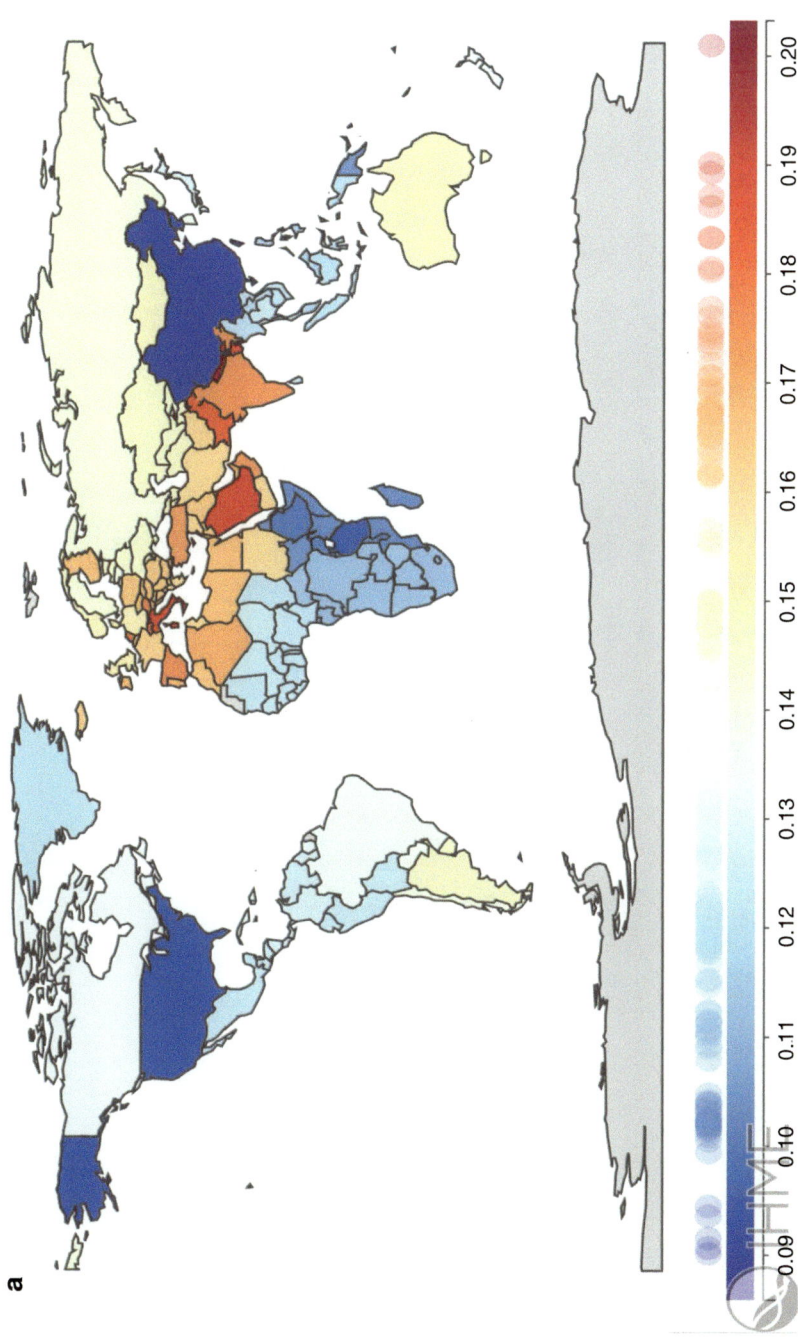

Fig. 1.2 (a) Global prevalence of migraine among men aged 15–49 years. (b) Global prevalence of migraine among women aged 15–49 years [18]

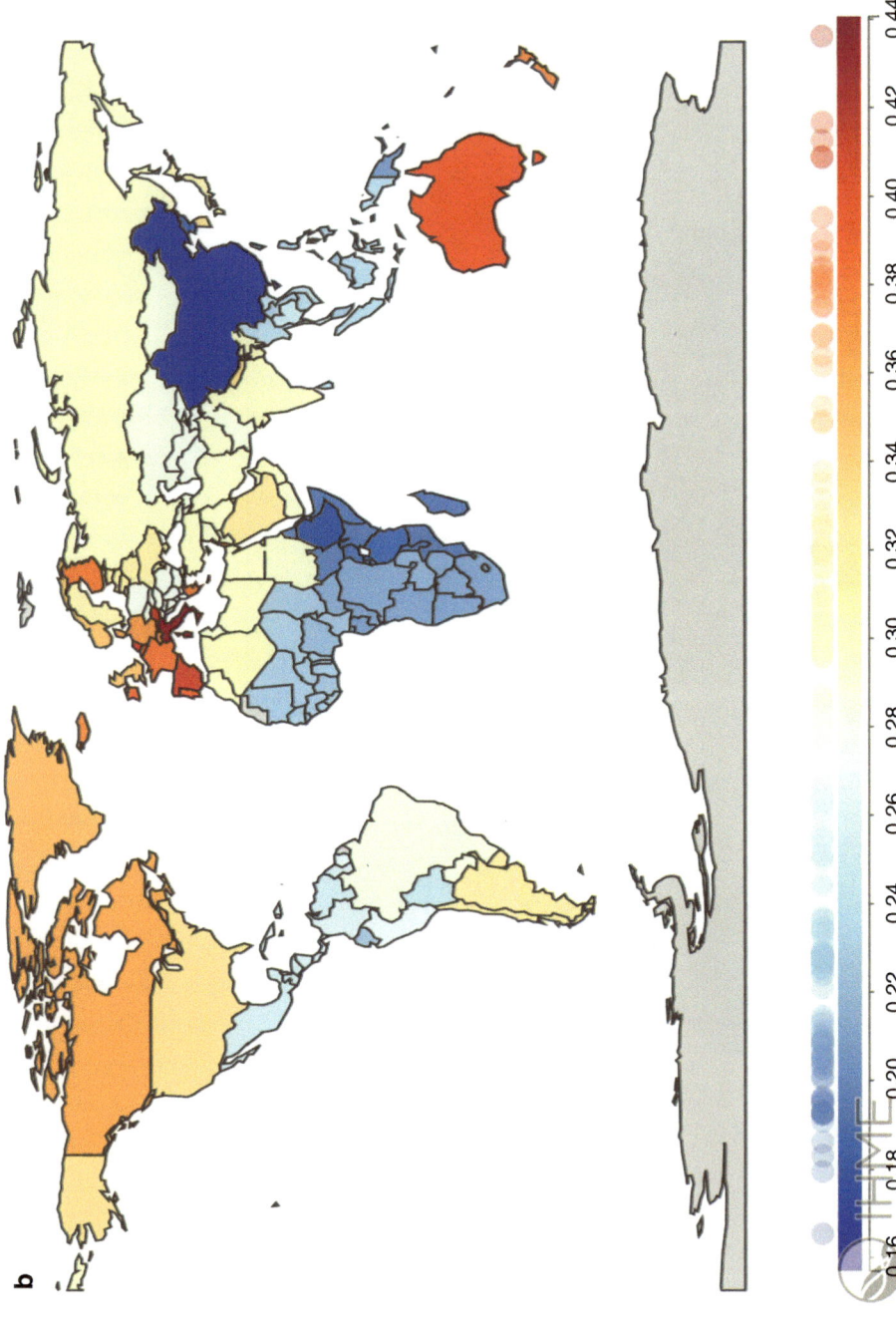

Fig. 1.2 (continued)

however consistently reported. Large population-based studies indicate that the 1-year prevalence and sex ratio are stable over time, with the numbers of men and women reporting migraine increasing in proportion to the population growth [12, 14, 16, 19].

1.2.1 Subtypes of Migraine

In both men and women, migraine without aura occurs about twice as often as migraine with aura, and the prevalence of migraine with aura is two to three times higher in women than men. Among men, the 1-year prevalence is within the range 0.6–3.4% with corresponding figures for women 1.9–7.4% [4, 16, 20–24]. A Danish study reported slightly higher figures for the lifetime prevalence of migraine with aura: 3.6% for men and 7.5% for women [25].

Chronic migraine accounts for about 8% of all migraine cases with prevalence estimates typically in the range of 1.4–2.2% [26]. Similar to the total migraine prevalence, the prevalence of chronic migraine peaks in the 40s in both sexes [27]. Chronic migraine is 4.7 times more common in women than men among young adults aged <30 years [28]. Thereafter, the prevalence is two to three times higher in women than in men, mirroring the sex ratio of the total migraine prevalence [27–29]. However, in the general population, chronic migraine is more prevalent within the total male migraine population than within the total female migraine population. This becomes specifically evident after the age of 40 when chronic migraine accounts for 9.9–11.7% of all male migraine cases as compared to 7.3–8.4% of all female migraine cases [27].

1.2.2 Incidence and Age at Onset

Age- and sex-specific incidence rates for migraine have been presented in both longitudinal and cross-sectional studies, although there is a dearth of longitudinal studies among adults [21, 30–33]. Common to all studies are the significant higher annual and cumulative incidence rates of migraine in women.

In a 12-year longitudinal Danish population-based study of 673 adults aged 25–64 years, the annual incidence rate of migraine was 8.1 per 1000 person-years with a male to female ratio of 1:6 [30]. Among both sexes, the incidence decreased significantly by age. The highest incidence was found among participants aged 25–34 years, with annual incidence rates of 6.5 per 1000 person-years for men and 22.8 per 1000 person-years for women.

Cross-sectional studies from the USA consistently report an earlier peak incidence in men [17, 34, 35]. The American Migraine Prevalence and Prevention (AMPP) study included more than 160,000 participants aged ≥12 years [17]. Migraine incidence peaked between the ages of 20 and 24 years in women (18.2 per

1000 person-years) and 15 and 19 years in men (6.2 per 1000 person-years) [17]. The median age at migraine onset was 24 years in men and 25 years in women. More than 75% of new-onset cases in men and more than 85% of new-onset female cases occurred *after* age 14 years. The cumulative lifetime incidence for migraine was significantly higher in women than men (43% vs. 18%). Another USA-based study that included younger participants (10–29 years) reported earlier migraine onset in men than in women for both migraine with aura (<5 years vs. 12–13 years) and without aura (11–12 years vs. 14–17 years) [34]. In contrast to men, new onset of migraine was relatively common among women in their late 20s. In both sexes, the incidence of migraine with aura peaked 3–5 years earlier than the incidence for migraine without aura.

A 30-year longitudinal study from Switzerland found that the cumulative incidence of migraine in men levelled off at age 35, whereas that in women continued to increase to age 50 [21]. The cumulative incidence of migraine in this prospective study was higher than estimates from the AMPP study: 50.7% in women and 20.7% in men.

A Danish study including 1136 twin pairs with a mean age of 36.6 years reported a later onset of migraine without aura in women than men (21.5 years vs. 16.5 years), while onset of migraine with aura did not differ significantly (21.8 years vs. 20.8 years) [36].

1.3 Natural History/Prognosis

Migraine is a fluctuating condition with periods of remission interposed by relapse; only about 35% of young adults with migraine continue to have intermittent attacks, while 20% continue to develop chronic migraine over 30-year follow-up [21].

Prospective studies of children and adolescents with migraine report higher remission rates in boys than in girls from childhood to young adulthood. In the long term, this sex difference seems to disappear, indicating that the capacity to have migraine remains in both men and women, with men being more likely to experience longer periods with remission [37–39].

To date, the longest prospective cohort of children with migraine is a 40-year follow-up study including 73 Swedish school children aged 7–15 years at baseline [11]. Before the age of 25 years, significantly more boys (34.9%) than girls (15.0%) were migraine-free. However, when the cohort reached around 50 years of age, 46% were migraine-free with no differences between the sexes.

A Finnish 25-year longitudinal study included 1185 children from the general population. The cohort was studied at three different ages: the age of 7, 14, and 32 years. Among the 7-year-olds, 4.0% had migraine (girls 3.7%, boys 4.3%, $p = 0.58$). At the age of 14 years, significantly more girls than boys had migraine (15% of girls and 7% boys, $p < 0.001$), and this sex difference remained significant when the cohort had reached the age of 32 years (22% girls vs. 8% boys, $p < 0.001$) [40]. Childhood migraine persisted into adulthood (from age 7–32) in 65% of women and 21% of men, while new onset of migraine occurred in 17% of the women and only 7% of men after childhood.

A population-based study of 1155 Turkish school children attending to the second to fifth school grade found that female sex was a significant risk factor for both development and persistence of migraine 6 years later, when the cohort had reached a mean age of 15.5 years [41]. During the 6 years, migraine prevalence among girls had increased from 9.9% to 21.5%. Corresponding figures for boys were 7.9% and 15.8%.

Studies from clinic populations display similar trends. An Italian clinic population including 64 children and adolescents (mean age 11.4 years, range 4–18) found that significantly more girls than boys had enduring migraine at 8-year follow-up (67% vs. 33%, $p < 0.05$) [42]. Similarly, a German study including 140 children and adolescents with mean age 17.6 years (range 11–26) at the time of follow-up found that female sex was a predictor for increased headache frequency from baseline 6.6 years earlier ($p = 0.04$) [43].

Longitudinal studies of adults present conflicting results. A French longitudinal study of 1250 employees aged 30–54 years at inclusion reported that retention or acquisition of a migraine diagnosis was more common in women than in men at 10-year follow-up [37]. In contrast, a Danish population-based study including 549 participants aged 25–64 years at inclusion reported that sex was not associated with poor outcome 12 years later [44].

Whether the prognosis differs between migraine with and without aura is uncertain, but studies suggest that men are more likely to experience longer periods with remission of migraine with aura. In a 10–20-year follow-up of a clinic sample including 81 patients aged 11–63 years, more men than women were attack-free for at least 1 year (46% vs. 29%) and 5 years (30.8% vs. 13.6%) [39]. In another clinic sample of 53 patients aged 12–66 years, a nonsignificant trend toward higher cessation rates for migraine with aura was found among men after 16-year follow-up (55% men vs. 31% women, $p = 0.17$) [38].

Regarding chronic migraine, population-based longitudinal studies show a more favorable prognosis for women. A recent German study reported that female sex was associated with remission of chronic headache (OR 2.29, 1.03–5.10) over a period of 3 years [45]. Similarly, in a US study of 1134 people with chronic migraine, the likelihood of remission increased with age for women, but not for men [46].

1.4 Phenotype

Studies consistently show that women report a longer duration of their migraine attacks compared to men [47–58], which may partly be due to the prolonged duration of menstrual attacks in women [59–61]. Other characteristics, such as pain intensity and attack frequency, do not differ among sexes in most studies [15, 19, 47, 48, 51, 52, 55, 57, 58, 62], with a few exceptions [4, 48]. Conversely, no studies report that men have more painful, longer-lasting, and more disabling migraine

attacks. The presence and severity of associated symptoms, such as photo- and phonophobia, nausea and vomiting, as well as cutaneous allodynia, are mostly reported
to be more prevalent in women [15, 19, 48, 50, 52, 56, 63]. In women, the clinical
features of migraine attacks vary significantly with age, while they show little alteration in men [48, 51, 56]. Sex differences in attack features have also been described
in children aged 11.7 years, with girls reporting longer duration and higher frequency of migraine [64].

These findings must however be interpreted with caution since most of the studies are based on retrospective self-report and retrospectively recorded migraine
symptoms may not correlate with those recorded prospectively. In addition, both
men and women rate men as less willing to report pain [65, 66].

1.5   The Impact of Migraine

Migraine causes a substantial amount of burden both to the affected individual and
to the society. The individual burden encompasses headache and associated symptoms, as well as limitations to activities at work and home and in social roles. The
societal burden involves indirect costs due to lost work time, underemployment, and
unemployment, as well as direct medical costs. The societal burden is further mediated by the high prevalence among working-age individuals.

The Global Burden of Disease (GBD) study 2016 ranks migraine as the fourth
leading cause of years lived with disability (YLDs) among women and number five
among men at all ages (Table 1.1). Among people aged 15–49, migraine is ranked
as number two among women and number three among men. Within each age
group, years lived with disability mirror the migraine prevalence and remain consistently higher in women than men (Fig. 1.3).

1.5.1   Individual Burden

Women consistently report a higher migraine-related disability and a longer period
of recovery after attacks than do men [4, 15, 52, 62, 67]. A US calculation from
1998 estimated that women spend 6 h in bed on average during migraine attacks
requiring bed rest, compared with 4.5 h in men [68]. On an annual basis, male
migraineurs were restricted to bed for 3.8 days and female migraineurs for 5.6 days.

The Migraine Disability Assessment (MIDAS) questionnaire is a frequently used
score to grade disability related to migraine [69]. This score consists of five items
and is graded 1–4, with 4 corresponding to severe disability and 1 to no/little disability. In the AMPP study, women were 1.34 times more likely than men to report

Table 1.1 Global ranking of years lived with disability (YLDs) by age and sex

	All ages	5–14 years	15–49 years	50–69 years
Women				
1	Low back pain	Skin diseases	Low back and neck pain	Low back and neck pain
2	Sense organ diseases	Iron-deficiency anemia	Migraine	Sense organ diseases
3	Skin diseases	Migraine	Depression	Depression
4	Migraine	Anxiety disorder	Skin diseases	Diabetes
5	Depression	Asthma	Iron-deficiency anemia	Migraine
6	Iron-deficiency anemia	Sense organ diseases	Other musculoskeletal disorders	Other musculoskeletal disorders
7	Other musculoskeletal disorders	Conduct disorder	Anxiety disorder	Osteoarthritis
8	Anxiety disorder	Congenital defect	Sense organ diseases	Skin diseases
9	Diabetes	Depression	Gynecological diseases	Oral disorders
10	Gynecological diseases	Neonatal preterm birth	Schizophrenia	Anxiety disorder
Men				
1	Low back pain	Skin diseases	Low back and neck pain	Low back and neck pain
2	Sense organ diseases	Iron-deficiency anemia	Skin diseases	Sense organ diseases
3	Skin diseases	Conduct disorder	Migraine	Diabetes
4	Depression	Sense organ diseases	Depression	Depression
5	Migraine	Asthma	Sense organ diseases	COPD
6	Diabetes	Autistic spectrum	Drug use disorder	Other musculoskeletal disorders
7	Iron-deficiency anemia	Anxiety disorder	Other musculoskeletal disorders	Falls
8	Other musculoskeletal disorders	Migraine	Anxiety disorder	Osteoarthritis
9	Anxiety disorder	Neonatal preterm birth	Diabetes	Oral disorders
10	Falls	Congenital defect	Alcohol use disorder	Migraine

Data from the Global Burden of Disease Study 2016 (GBD 2016) [18]

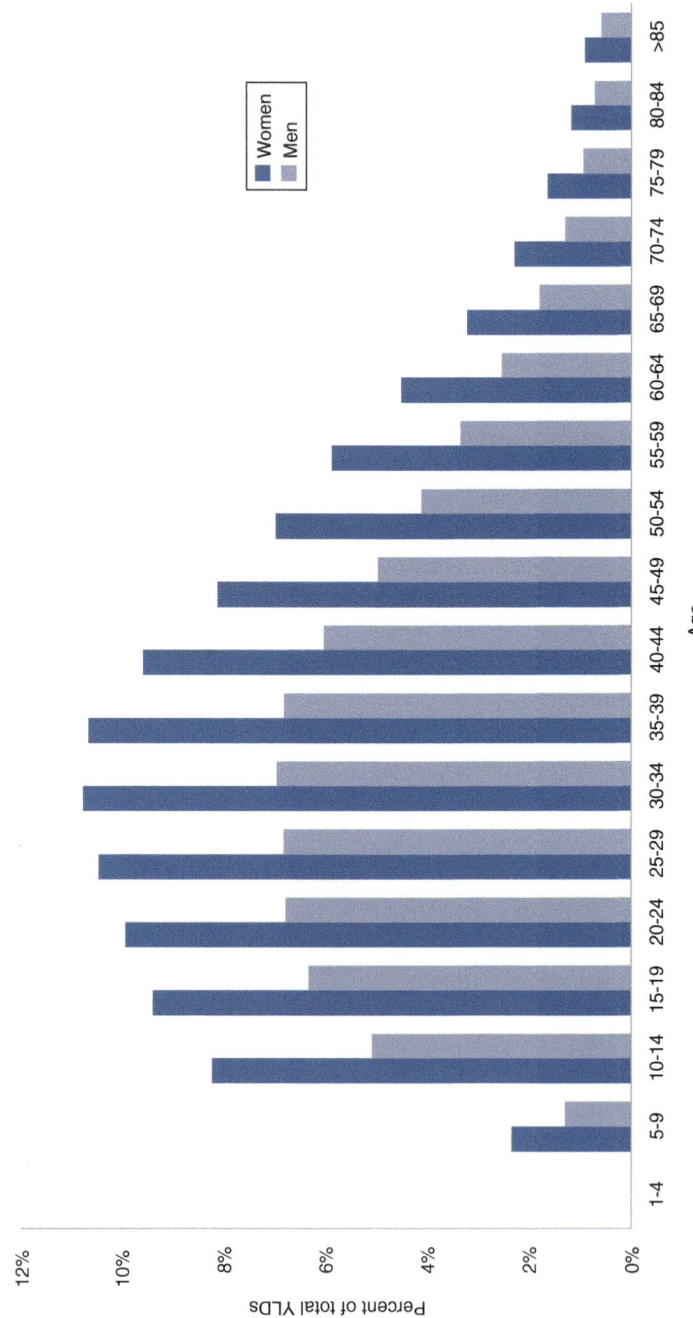

Fig. 1.3 Years Lived with Disability (YLDs) by age and sex. Data from the Global Burden of Disease Study 2016 (GBD 2016) [18]

MIDAS grade 4 [15]. Examination of the individual MIDAS items revealed that female migraineurs were significantly more likely to report inability or reduced productivity in household work due to headache and to miss family or social activities. No significant sex difference was observed in relation to missed workdays or days with reduced productivity at work. This contrasts with an older US study reporting that women lost on average 8.3 workdays per year due to severe headache, whereas the corresponding figure for men was 3.8 days [70]. European studies confirm the higher migraine-related disability in women, although comparable studies presenting the individual MIDAS items are lacking [4, 52, 71].

The HALT index (Headache-Attributed Lost Time index) is another score that assesses the impact of migraine in terms of lost useful time [72]. This index captures the number of lost days due to headache over 3 months in three categories: days of paid work, household, and social days. A European study including migraineurs from nine different countries reported that 15.8% of female migraineurs lost more than 20 days in total due to migraine during the preceding 3 months, compared to 9.9% of men [73]. Women reported higher numbers of lost days in all categories. This finding is however not consistent across different countries and cultures. In Lithuania no significant differences among male and female migraineurs were found in all three categories measured by the HALT index [58]. In India, women lost more days in total and days of household than men, but no sex difference was found in the number of lost workdays [74]. In the low-income countries Nepal and Ethiopia, women lost significantly more household worktime than men, while the reverse was so for paid worktime [57, 75]. However, in Nepal men lost significantly more days in total than did women [57].

Whether a sex difference in migraine-related disability also exists among children and adolescents is uncertain. In a clinical sample of 4121 patients aged 1–21 years (mean 11.7 ± 3.6), girls had significantly higher average pediatric MIDAS score compared to boys [64]. Two other studies among children and adolescents could however not detect a difference in the Pediatric MIDAS [41, 76].

1.5.2 Societal Burden

A 2012 study estimated that migraine costs the European society more than 111 billion euros annually, resulting in a mean per person annual cost of € 1222 (95% CI 1055–1389) [77]. More than 90% of these costs are indirect, i.e., costs related to work absenteeism, loss of productivity at work, and early retirement. Sex-specific estimates were not presented in this and other recent studies dealing with costs [78].

US data from 1999 suggest that female migraineurs account for about 80% of the direct and indirect costs associated with migraine [68]. The annual economic loss attributable to migraine-related absenteeism and reduced productivity was four times higher in women than men (USD 2660.3 million for men and USD 10,688.8 million for women) [68]. Even these high costs were probably an underestimate since they did not consider unemployment and underemployment due to migraine.

The direct annual costs, i.e., costs associated with treatment, such as physician office visit, emergency department visits, inpatient care, and prescription of drugs, were also higher for women than for men (97.32 USD vs. 89.97 USD).

In conclusion, migraine is predominantly a female disorder during all years following puberty. The maximum sex difference is between age 30–45, when the migraine prevalence peaks in both men and women. Migraine is ranked as the second most common cause of disability among women aged 15–49 years and the third leading cause among men at this age category. Women have a longer duration of attacks and report a higher migraine-related disability, while men are more likely to experience longer periods of remission.

References

1. Headache Classification Subcommittee of the International Headache Society. The International Classification of Headache Disorders, 3rd edition (beta version). Cephalalgia. 2013;33:629–808.
2. Goadsby PJ, Holland PR, Martins-Oliveira M, et al. Pathophysiology of migraine: a disorder of sensory processing. Physiol Rev. 2017;97:553–622.
3. Rasmussen BK, Olesen J. Migraine with aura and migraine without aura: an epidemiological study. Cephalalgia. 1992;12:221–8. discussion 186.
4. Radtke A, Neuhauser H. Prevalence and burden of headache and migraine in Germany. Headache. 2009;49:79–89.
5. Russell MB, Rasmussen BK, Thorvaldsen P, Olesen J. Prevalence and sex-ratio of the subtypes of migraine. Int J Epidemiol. 1995;24(3):612–8.
6. Charles AC, Baca SM. Cortical spreading depression and migraine. Nat Rev Neurol. 2013;9:637–44.
7. Mortimer MJ, Kay J, Jaron A. Childhood migraine in general practice: clinical features and characteristics. Cephalalgia. 1992;12:238–43. discussion 186.
8. Milovanovic M, Jarebinski M, Martinovic Z. Prevalence of primary headaches in children from Belgrade, Serbia. Eur J Paediatr Neurol. 2007;11:136–41.
9. Isik U, Ersu RH, Ay P, et al. Prevalence of headache and its association with sleep disorders in children. Pediatr Neurol. 2007;36:146–51.
10. Stovner LJ, Zwart JA, Hagen K, et al. Epidemiology of headache in Europe. Eur J Neurol. 2006;13:333–45.
11. Bille B. A 40-year follow-up of school children with migraine. Cephalalgia. 1997;17:488–91. discussion 87.
12. Stewart WF, Lipton RB, Celentano DD, et al. Prevalence of migraine headache in the United States. Relation to age, income, race, and other sociodemographic factors. JAMA. 1992;267:64–9.
13. Stovner L, Hagen K, Jensen R, et al. The global burden of headache: a documentation of headache prevalence and disability worldwide. Cephalalgia. 2007;27:193–210.
14. Lipton RB, Bigal ME, Diamond M, et al. Migraine prevalence, disease burden, and the need for preventive therapy. Neurology. 2007;68:343–9.
15. Buse DC, Loder EW, Gorman JA, et al. Sex differences in the prevalence, symptoms, and associated features of migraine, probable migraine and other severe headache: results of the American Migraine Prevalence and Prevention (AMPP) Study. Headache. 2013;53:1278–99.
16. Linde M, Stovner LJ, Zwart JA, et al. Time trends in the prevalence of headache disorders. The Nord-Trondelag Health Studies (HUNT 2 and HUNT 3). Cephalalgia. 2011;31:585–96.

17. Stewart WF, Wood C, Reed ML, et al. Cumulative lifetime migraine incidence in women and men. Cephalalgia. 2008;28:1170–8.
18. Institute for Health Metrics and Evaluation (IHME). **GBD Compare**. Seattle, WA: IHME, University of Washington, 2016. Available from http://vizhub.healthdata.org/gbd-compare. Accessed 20th December 2017.
19. Lipton RB, Stewart WF, Diamond S, et al. Prevalence and burden of migraine in the United States: data from the American Migraine Study II. Headache. 2001;41:646–57.
20. Winkler AS, Dent W, Stelzhammer B, et al. Prevalence of migraine headache in a rural area of northern Tanzania: a community-based door-to-door survey. Cephalalgia. 2010;30:582–92.
21. Merikangas KR, Cui L, Richardson AK, et al. Magnitude, impact, and stability of primary headache subtypes: 30 year prospective Swiss cohort study. BMJ. 2011;343:d5076.
22. Ferrante T, Castellini P, Abrignani G, et al. The PACE study: past-year prevalence of migraine in Parma's adult general population. Cephalalgia. 2012;32:358–65.
23. Ertas M, Baykan B, Orhan EK, et al. One-year prevalence and the impact of migraine and tension-type headache in Turkey: a nationwide home-based study in adults. J Headache Pain. 2012;13:147–57.
24. Silva Junior AA, Bigal M, Vasconcelos LP, et al. Prevalence and burden of headaches as assessed by the health family program. Headache. 2012;52:483–90.
25. Russell MB, Rasmussen BK, Thorvaldsen P, et al. Prevalence and sex-ratio of the subtypes of migraine. Int J Epidemiol. 1995;24:612–8.
26. Natoli JL, Manack A, Dean B, et al. Global prevalence of chronic migraine: a systematic review. Cephalalgia. 2010;30:599–609.
27. Buse DC, Manack AN, Fanning KM, et al. Chronic migraine prevalence, disability, and sociodemographic factors: results from the American Migraine Prevalence and Prevention Study. Headache. 2012;52:1456–70.
28. Katsarava Z, Dzagnidze A, Kukava M, et al. Primary headache disorders in the Republic of Georgia: prevalence and risk factors. Neurology. 2009;73:1796–803.
29. da Silva A Jr, Costa EC, Gomes JB, et al. Chronic headache and comorbidities: a two-phase, population-based, cross-sectional study. Headache. 2010;50:1306–12.
30. Lyngberg AC, Rasmussen BK, Jorgensen T, et al. Incidence of primary headache: a Danish epidemiologic follow-up study. Am J Epidemiol. 2005;161:1066–73.
31. Breslau N, Davis GC, Schultz LR, et al. Joint 1994 Wolff Award Presentation. Migraine and major depression: a longitudinal study. Headache. 1994;34:387–93.
32. Breslau N, Chilcoat HD, Andreski P. Further evidence on the link between migraine and neuroticism. Neurology. 1996;47:663–7.
33. Swartz KL, Pratt LA, Armenian HK, et al. Mental disorders and the incidence of migraine headaches in a community sample: results from the Baltimore Epidemiologic Catchment area follow-up study. Arch Gen Psychiatry. 2000;57:945–50.
34. Stewart WF, Linet MS, Celentano DD, et al. Age- and sex-specific incidence rates of migraine with and without visual aura. Am J Epidemiol. 1991;134:1111–20.
35. Stang PE, Yanagihara PA, Swanson JW, et al. Incidence of migraine headache: a population-based study in Olmsted County, Minnesota. Neurology. 1992;42:1657–62.
36. Ulrich V, Gervil M, Fenger K, et al. The prevalence and characteristics of migraine in twins from the general population. Headache. 1999;39:173–80.
37. Nachit-Ouinekh F, Dartigues JF, Chrysostome V, et al. Evolution of migraine after a 10-year follow-up. Headache. 2005;45:1280–7.
38. Eriksen MK, Thomsen LL, Russell MB. Prognosis of migraine with aura. Cephalalgia. 2004;24:18–22.
39. Cologno D, Torelli P, Manzoni GC. Migraine with aura: a review of 81 patients at 10-20 years' follow-up. Cephalalgia. 1998;18:690–6.
40. Sillanpaa M, Saarinen MM. Long term outcome of childhood onset headache: a prospective community study. Cephalalgia. 2018;38:1159.

41. Ozge A, Sasmaz T, Cakmak SE, et al. Epidemiological-based childhood headache natural history study: after an interval of six years. Cephalalgia. 2010;30:703–12.
42. Guidetti V, Galli F. Evolution of headache in childhood and adolescence: an 8-year follow-up. Cephalalgia. 1998;18:449–54.
43. Kienbacher C, Wober C, Zesch HE, et al. Clinical features, classification and prognosis of migraine and tension-type headache in children and adolescents: a long-term follow-up study. Cephalalgia. 2006;26:820–30.
44. Lyngberg AC, Rasmussen BK, Jorgensen T, et al. Prognosis of migraine and tension-type headache: a population-based follow-up study. Neurology. 2005;65:580–5.
45. Henning V, Katsarava Z, Obermann M, et al. Remission of chronic headache: rates, potential predictors and the role of medication, follow-up results of the German Headache Consortium (GHC) Study. Cephalalgia. 2018;38:551.
46. Scher AI, Stewart WF, Ricci JA, et al. Factors associated with the onset and remission of chronic daily headache in a population-based study. Pain. 2003;106:81–9.
47. Kelman L. Pain characteristics of the acute migraine attack. Headache. 2006;46:942–53.
48. Bolay H, Ozge A, Saginc P, et al. Gender influences headache characteristics with increasing age in migraine patients. Cephalalgia. 2015;35:792–800.
49. Kallela M, Wessman M, Farkkila M, et al. Clinical characteristics of migraine in a population-based twin sample: similarities and differences between migraine with and without aura. Cephalalgia. 1999;19:151–8.
50. Murtaza M, Kisat M, Daniel H, et al. Classification and clinical features of headache disorders in Pakistan: a retrospective review of clinical data. PLoS One. 2009;4:e5827.
51. Wober-Bingol C, Wober C, Karwautz A, et al. Clinical features of migraine: a cross-sectional study in patients aged three to sixty-nine. Cephalalgia. 2004;24:12–7.
52. Steiner TJ, Scher AI, Stewart WF, et al. The prevalence and disability burden of adult migraine in England and their relationships to age, gender and ethnicity. Cephalalgia. 2003;23:519–27.
53. Franconi F, Finocchi C, Allais G, et al. Gender and triptan efficacy: a pooled analysis of three double-blind, randomized, crossover, multicenter, Italian studies comparing frovatriptan vs. other triptans. Neurol Sci. 2014;35(Suppl 1):99–105.
54. Kelman L, Harper SQ, Hu X, et al. Treatment response and tolerability of frovatriptan in patients reporting short- or long-duration migraines at baseline. Curr Med Res Opin. 2010;26:2097–104.
55. Russell MB, Rasmussen BK, Fenger K, et al. Migraine without aura and migraine with aura are distinct clinical entities: a study of four hundred and eighty-four male and female migraineurs from the general population. Cephalalgia. 1996;16:239–45.
56. Ozge A, Uluduz D, Selekler M, et al. Gender differences in older adults with chronic migraine in Turkey. Geriatr Gerontol Int. 2015;15:652–8.
57. Manandhar K, Risal A, Linde M, et al. The burden of headache disorders in Nepal: estimates from a population-based survey. J Headache Pain. 2015;17:3.
58. Rastenyte D, Mickeviciene D, Stovner LJ, et al. Prevalence and burden of headache disorders in Lithuania and their public-health and policy implications: a population-based study within the Eurolight Project. J Headache Pain. 2017;18:53.
59. Vetvik KG, Benth JS, MacGregor EA, et al. Menstrual versus non-menstrual attacks of migraine without aura in women with and without menstrual migraine. Cephalalgia. 2015;35:1261–8.
60. MacGregor EA, Victor TW, Hu X, et al. Characteristics of menstrual vs nonmenstrual migraine: a post hoc, within-woman analysis of the usual-care phase of a nonrandomized menstrual migraine clinical trial. Headache. 2010;50:528–38.
61. Pinkerman B, Holroyd K. Menstrual and nonmenstrual migraines differ in women with menstrually-related migraine. Cephalalgia. 2010;30:1187–94.
62. Henry P, Auray JP, Gaudin AF, et al. Prevalence and clinical characteristics of migraine in France. Neurology. 2002;59:232–7.
63. d'Agostino VC, Francia E, Licursi V, et al. Clinical and personality features of allodynic migraine. Neurol Sci. 2010;31(Suppl 1):S159–61.

64. Slater S, Crawford MJ, Kabbouche MA, et al. Effects of gender and age on paediatric headache. Cephalalgia. 2009;29:969–73.
65. Hansen JM, Goadsby PJ, Charles AC. Variability of clinical features in attacks of migraine with aura. Cephalalgia. 2016;36:216–24.
66. Robinson ME, Riley JL III, Myers CD, et al. Gender role expectations of pain: relationship to sex differences in pain. J Pain. 2001;2:251–7.
67. Stewart WF, Shechter A, Lipton RB. Migraine heterogeneity. Disability, pain intensity, and attack frequency and duration. Neurology. 1994;44:S24–39.
68. Hu XH, Markson LE, Lipton RB, et al. Burden of migraine in the United States: disability and economic costs. Arch Intern Med. 1999;159:813–8.
69. Stewart WF, Lipton RB, Kolodner KB, et al. Validity of the Migraine Disability Assessment (MIDAS) score in comparison to a diary-based measure in a population sample of migraine sufferers. Pain. 2000;88:41–52.
70. Stewart WF, Lipton RB, Simon D. Work-related disability: results from the American migraine study. Cephalalgia. 1996;16:231–8. discussion 15.
71. Henry P, Michel P, Brochet B, et al. A nationwide survey of migraine in France: prevalence and clinical features in adults. GRIM. Cephalalgia. 1992;12:229–37. discussion 186.
72. Steiner T. The HALT and HART indices. J Headache Pain. 2007;8(Suppl 1):S22–5.
73. Steiner TJ, Stovner LJ, Katsarava Z, et al. The impact of headache in Europe: principal results of the Eurolight project. J Headache Pain. 2014;15:31.
74. Rao GN, Kulkarni GB, Gururaj G, et al. The burden attributable to headache disorders in India: estimates from a community-based study in Karnataka State. J Headache Pain. 2015;16:94.
75. Zebenigus M, Tekle-Haimanot R, Worku DK, et al. The burden of headache disorders in Ethiopia: national estimates from a population-based door-to-door survey. J Headache Pain. 2017;18:58.
76. Akyol A, Kiylioglu N, Aydin I, et al. Epidemiology and clinical characteristics of migraine among school children in the Menderes region. Cephalalgia. 2007;27:781–7.
77. Linde M, Gustavsson A, Stovner LJ, et al. The cost of headache disorders in Europe: the Eurolight project. Eur J Neurol. 2012;19:703–11.
78. Messali A, Sanderson JC, Blumenfeld AM, et al. Direct and indirect costs of chronic and episodic migraine in the United States: a web-based survey. Headache. 2016;56:306–22.

Chapter 2
Cardiovascular Risk of Migraine in Men and Women

L. Al-Hassany, K. A. Linstra, G. M. Terwindt, and Antoinette Maassen van den Brink

2.1 Introduction

The association of migraine, particularly migraine with aura—characterized by focal neurological symptoms—and different forms of cardiovascular disease and cardiovascular mortality has been a topic of much debate [1]. However, with recent advances made in this field, migraine with aura has now been acknowledged as an established risk factor for (subclinical) ischemic lesions in the brain and white matter lesions [2]. Moreover, a broader range of ischemic vascular disorders, including myocardial ischemia, has been studied. Although migraine mainly affects young women and the majority of data available on an association with cardiovascular disease is based on females, an association between migraine and cardiovascular disease has also been observed in men [2]. The assumption that the presence or absence of cardiovascular disease influences the additional cardiovascular risk associated with migraine therefore may have consequences for the choices of pharmacological antimigraine treatment [3].

L. Al-Hassany · A. Maassen van den Brink (✉)
Divisionof Pharmacology and Vascular Medicine, Department of Internal Medicine, Erasmus University Medical Center, Rotterdam, The Netherlands
e-mail: a.vanharen-maassenvandenbrink@erasmusmc.nl

K. A. Linstra
Division of Pharmacology and Vascular Medicine, Department of Internal Medicine, Erasmus University Medical Center, Rotterdam, The Netherlands

Department of Neurology, Leiden University Medical Center, Leiden, The Netherlands
e-mail: k.linstra@erasmusmc.nl

G. M. Terwindt
Department of Neurology, Leiden University Medical Center, Leiden, The Netherlands
e-mail: G.M.Terwindt@lumc.nl

© Springer Nature Switzerland AG 2019
A. Maassen van den Brink, E. A. MacGregor (eds.), *Gender and Migraine*, Headache, https://doi.org/10.1007/978-3-030-02988-3_2

   This chapter will touch upon various topics concerning cardiovascular disease and migraine in both men and women, including its possible pathophysiological mechanisms, risk factors, clinical consequences, and unanswered questions [4].

2.2   Epidemiological Outcomes of Cardiovascular Risks in Migraineurs

Several studies have investigated the association between migraine and various forms of cardiovascular disease. Particularly migraine with aura has been found to be associated with an increased risk of vascular events, including ischemic and hemorrhagic stroke, myocardial infarction, and angina pectoris [5–8].

   The most relevant cohort studies have been summarized in Table 2.1, which has been modified from Linstra et al. [5]. We also recommend the overview of meta-analyses concerning the association of migraine and ischemic stroke, migraine and hemorrhagic stroke, as well as migraine and vascular disease provided by Sacco and Bushnell [6]. Moreover, Hu et al. [4] recently published an updated meta-analysis, which focuses primarily on migraine and the risk of stroke.

   Besides the fact that migraine is positively associated with cardio- and cerebrovascular disease, it is also associated with structural cardiac anomalies. Right-to-left shunts are more prevalent in migraineurs, which include the patent foramen ovale (PFO), atrial septal defects, and pulmonary right-to-left shunt. Prevalent structural anomalies that are not related to shunting include mitral valve prolapse, atrial septal aneurysm, and congenital heart disease [18].

2.3   Pathophysiological Mechanisms of Migraine and Cardiovascular Disease

Understanding the origin of migraine aids in the understanding of the potential association with cardiovascular disease and thus in the clinical assessment of the patient. Also, a better comprehension contributes to an improved adjustment between the need for treatment and the actual choice of pharmacological treatment in individuals who are or may be at increased risk for cardiovascular disease. Identifying high-risk patients implies the need for diagnostic vigilance as well [2].

   Moreover, an increasing understanding of the link between migraine and cardiovascular disease will help to formulate relevant, unanswered research questions. Therefore, this chapter reviews current theories about the link between migraine and cardiovascular disease, with special emphasis on the role of gender in this relation.

   Bigal et al. [2] proposed different conceptual mechanisms: (1) an association between migraine and cardiovascular disease may not exist due to bias, or the

Table 2.1 Cohort studies investigating the association of migraine and cardiovascular disease (other than stroke)

Author	Study type	Population (n =)	Age range	Follow-up duration	Migraine type (diagnosis)	CVD specification	Associated risk (95% CI)
Kurth et al. [9]	Prospective cohort (follow-up >20 years)	Women (115,541)	25–42	240 months	All migraine (self-reported physician's diagnosis)	Major CVD (MI, all stroke types, fatal CVD) MI CV mortality	HR 1.50 (1.33–1.69) HR 1.39 (1.18–1.64) HR 1.37 (1.02–1.83)
Wang et al. [10]	Retrospective cohort	Both (23,082)	18–45	29.2 months	All migraine (medical records)	IHD	HR 2.50 (1.78–3.52)
Bigal et al. [11]	Case control	Both (11,345)		5 years	All migraine MA MO (validated questionnaire IHS2 criteria)	MI MI MI	OR 2.19 (1.73–2.77) OR 2.99 (2.27–3.95) OR 1.80 (1.39–2.34)
Gudmundsson et al. [12]	Prospective cohort	Both (18,725)	33–81	25.9 years	All MA MO (interview IHS 2 criteria)	CV mortality CV mortality CV mortality	HR 1.19 (1.07–1.32) HR 1.27 (1.13–1.43) HR 1.10 (0.91–1.34)
Schürks et al. [7]	Meta-analysis	Both	Any		Heterogenous	MI CV mortality	Pooled 1.12 (0.95–1.32) Pooled 1.03 (0.79–1.34)
Kurth et al. [13]	Prospective cohort (FU 16 years)	Men (20,084)	40–84	15.7 years	All migraine (self-report migraine attack)	Major CVD (MI, stroke, fatal CVD) CV mortality	HR 1.12 (0.84–1.50) HR 1.07 (0.80–1.43)

(continued)

Table 2.1 (continued)

Author	Study type	Population (n =)	Age range	Follow-up duration	Migraine type (diagnosis)	CVD specification	Associated risk (95% CI)
Ahmed et al. [14]	Retrospective cohort	Women (873)	Any	4.4 years	All migraine (self-report questionnaire)	CV event / CV mortality	HR 1.21 (0.93–1.58) / HR 1.16 (0.20–6.7)
Velentgas et al. [15]	Retrospective cohort	Both (260,822)	Any	1.36 person-years, for a total of 353,190 person-years	All migraine (triptan use or based on medical record)	MI / CV mortality	RR 0.96 (0.80–1.15) / RR 0.60 (0.33–1.09)
Hall et al. [16]	Retrospective cohort	Both (140,814)	Any		All migraine (medical record)	MI / CV mortality	HR 1.15 (0.96–1.38) / HR 0.93 (0.76–1.13)
Sternfeld et al. [17]	Retrospective cohort	Both (79,588); Men; Women; Men; Women; Men; Women; Men; Women	Any <40		All migraine; Frequent unilateral headaches with nausea or affected vision; Self-reported physician's diagnosis or treatment; Frequent unilateral headaches with nausea or affected vision; Self-reported physician's diagnosis or treatment	MI; MI; MI; MI; MI; MI; MI; MI	RR 0.8 (0.5–1.2); RR 0.7 (0.4–1.0); RR 1.2 (0.7–1.9); RR 1.4 (0.9–2.1); RR 0.3 (0.1–2.4); RR 1.5 (0.5–5.1); RR 0.6 (0.1–4.4); RR 2.1 (0.5–9.5)

CV cardiovascular, CVD cardiovascular disease, HR hazard ratio, MA migraine with aura, MI myocardial infarction, MO migraine without aura, OR odds ratio, RR relative risk
Modified from Linstra et al. [5]

diseases coexist in a noncausal manner (mechanism A, although this of course is not a real mechanism); (2) a unidirectional causal relationship exists between migraine (or its consequences on the vasculature, according to Sacco et al. [1]) and cardiovascular disease (mechanism B); (3) migraine and cardiovascular disease share the same environmental risk factors (mechanism C); and (4) migraine and cardiovascular disease have common genetic or biologic risk factors (mechanism D) [1, 2]. Sacco et al. [1] added additional possible mechanisms to these concepts, which may partly overlap with the mechanisms mentioned above: at least one comorbid condition with migraine is responsible for the elevated risk for cardiovascular disease (mechanism E), and a shared underlying disease leads to both migraine and cardiovascular disease (mechanism F).

To explain the relationship between migraine and cardiovascular events, it is of importance to understand the mechanisms involved in migraine. Three major theories for the pathophysiology of migraine have been described in literature, including the vascular theory, the neurovascular theory, and the theory of cortical spreading depression (CSD) [19]. Currently, it seems most likely that migraine is not an exclusively vascular nor an exclusively neuronal disorder. Thus, the neurovascular system seems involved in the generation of migraine attacks. Dysregulation of the neurovascular system during a migraine attack may be a manifestation, as well as a cause of cerebrovascular damage in migraine patients. Indeed, subclinical damage, presented as white matter hyperintensities and silent brain lesions on MRI, is found to be more prevalent in patients with migraine, especially in female migraineurs [20]. The connection of migraine with non-cerebral vascular damage, such as coronary heart disease, is more difficult to comprehend. To understand this relation, a certain systemic "vascular vulnerability" [18] would be likely (see above, mechanism C/D). Migraine could be regarded as an expression of this underlying condition which, when combined with other modifiers of vascular health, may lead to a synergistic increase in CVD risk. This hypothesis could explain the multiplicative risk seen in young female migraineurs who smoke and use oral contraceptives [21]. Ongoing research is aiming to define this vascular vulnerability. Below, we will discuss certain factors that may contribute to the vascular vulnerability in migraine.

2.3.1 Endothelial Dysfunction

The systemic disorder "endothelial dysfunction," characterized by, among other factors, impaired nitric oxide (NO) bioavailability, has been named as the "ultimate risk of the risk factors" [22]. Unfortunately, studies on the vascular reactivity in migraine patients have resulted in inconsistent results and have not led to definite conclusions yet—possibly due to the heterogeneity between these studies. However, several studies support the idea of a deterioration of arterial function in migraine [23]. Currently available methods, such as transcranial Doppler during breath-holding [24], peripheral plethysmography by EndoPAT, or measurement of local thermal hyperemia [25], to measure the peripheral endothelial function might lead to a screening method to estimate the cerebral or peripheral endothelial function [26, 27]. Obviously, all of these methods have their limitations and do not comprehensively measure all aspects of endothelial function.

Thus, novel developments on the assessment of endothelial function are awaited with interest.

2.3.2   Platelet Abnormalities

The hypothesis of migraine being caused by a primary abnormality of the behavior of platelets has been put forward in 1978 [28]. Nowadays, no consensus has been reached about the exact role of the platelets in the pathogenesis of migraine, although data suggest a pivotal and predisposing role of serotonin (5-hydroxytryptamine, 5-HT) availability in migraineurs [29]. Abnormalities in spontaneous platelet activation and aggregation have been observed and confirmed, caused by changes in the expression of fibrinogen receptors, platelet glycoprotein IIb, and the 5-HT_2 serotonin receptors [29–32]. Moreover, several pharmacological studies with aspirin, 5-HT-releasing agents, and serotonin uptake inhibitors have supported the involvement of platelet aggregation in the pathogenesis of migraine [29].

2.3.3   Microemboli

The role of microemboli in the pathogenesis of migraine and associated vascular disease has been controversial, due to the conflicting evidence of the pathophysiological importance of PFO in migraine. About a decade ago, it was assessed whether closure of the PFO would prevent subclinical microemboli and metabolites (e.g., serotonin) to bypass the pulmonary circulation via this right-to-left shunt [27, 33]. These small studies assessing the effect of PFO closure on migraine showed several biases, including the use of aspirin and blinding issues in the trials [34]. The results of the randomized clinical trial *Migraine Intervention with STARFlex Technology (MIST)* did not support closure of the PFO to prevent migraine attacks with aura [35].

2.3.4   Shared Genetic Markers

The identification of susceptibility genes for migraine is a challenging area, mainly due to the contribution of multiple and potentially interacting genetic loci. Moreover, environmental factors play a confounding role [36]. Despite the difficulties in assigning genes responsible of an increase of the risk for migraine, it seems evident that genetic diversity is an important factor in determining the risk for the development of migraine. Common forms of migraine (with or without aura) have been linked to several loci, showing enrichment for genes expressed in vascular and smooth muscle tissues [37]. Winsvold et al. [38] determined the genetic overlap between migraine and coronary artery disease by performing analyses based on three large GWAS meta-analyses of migraine and coronary artery disease. The authors confirm previous reports that migraine and CAD share genetic risk loci in excess of what would be expected by chance and highlight one shared risk locus encoding the *PHACTR1* gene [38], encoding for the protein phosphatase and actin regulator 1, a protein phosphatase 1 binding protein that is highly expressed in the brain.

2.4 Gender Differences in Migraine and Cardiovascular Risk

Limited direct estimates and comparisons of the cardiovascular risk in male versus female migraine patients are available. Moreover, given the fact that migraine is approximately three times more common in women than in men, male populations with the same size as female populations may have lower statistical power [39]. Therefore, it is yet impossible to draw a firm conclusion on whether the cardiovascular risk is higher in females with migraine compared to male migraine patients [40].

Studies on the cardiovascular risk in men with migraine are rare, but their results are compatible with data evidencing an increased risk for CVD in women with migraine. A large prospective cohort study with 22,071 participants by Kurth et al. [13] of (initially) healthy middle-aged men showed a 24% increased risk of major cardiovascular risk factors and a 42% increased risk for nonfatal myocardial infarction. Furthermore, insignificant correlations have been found with increased risks of ischemic stroke, death from ischemic cardiovascular disease, or coronary revascularization [13]. These results are in line with findings of an older study by Cook et al. [41], who evaluated migraine as an independent risk factor and adjusted for other risk factors. The comparison between both genders did not show an increased significant risk for major coronary heart disease (nonfatal myocardial infarction or fatal coronary heart diseases) and total coronary heart diseases (major coronary heart disease plus angina and coronary revascularization) [42].

2.4.1 The Role of Hormones

Fluctuations in sex hormone levels seem to be associated with an increased sensitivity for migraine [43]. (Changing levels of) estrogens may enhance the susceptibility in females to migraine by increasing the earlier mentioned cortical excitability, as well as via (neuro)vascular mechanisms [44]. Studies of the effects of estrogen on seizure threshold support this hypothesis [40]. The sex hormones (i.e., estrogen, progesterone/progestin, testosterone) have a major influence on vascular health [43]. Interestingly, while migraine attacks are well documented to be most prominent around menstruation [43], a number of case series and case reports have also implicated a relationship between the cardiac symptoms and the menstrual period [45–47].

Unfortunately, the evidence thus far is scarce, and mechanisms implied in a potential relationship between migraine, cardiovascular disease, and hormones should be investigated in more detail.

2.5 Biomarkers and Markers of Subclinical Vascular Disease

A systematic review by Tietjen et al. [48] indicated a number of positive vascular biomarker studies in migraine populations, including some involving novel bio-markers such as endothelial microparticles and endothelial precursor cells [48]. However, it should be kept in mind that no biomarkers investigated to date have the sensitivity and specificity to diagnose migraine outside of its clinical context. A number of positive vascular biomarker studies in migraine populations lend insight into possible pathophysiological mechanisms by which migraine may be associated with cardiovascular disease.

Recently, an association between elevated selected vascular disease biomarkers and migraine, particularly in the high-risk groups (women with aura), was reported [49]. Specifically, it was aura (not headache, frequency of attacks, and duration since onset) that strengthened the relationship with plasma concentrations of the biomarkers fibrinogen, high-sensitivity C-reactive protein (hs-CRP), von Willebrand factor antigen (vWF Ag), and D-dimer [49].

Subclinical markers of vascular disease have also been suggested to be altered in patients with migraine. As a part of the *Atherosclerosis Risk in Communities Study*, retinal microvascular signs were assessed among middle-aged persons with migraine. After correcting for age, sex, ethnicity, and cardiovascular risk factors, migraine has been found to be associated with (signs of) retinopathy—with stronger associations in the subset patients without a history of diabetes or hypertension [2, 50]. The vascular shared mechanism may be an endotheliopathy and not classic atherosclerosis as was suggested by Stam et al. [51].

2.6 Consequences for the Clinical Practice
and for Healthcare Professionals

Despite the convincing evidence of the relationship between migraine (mainly with aura) and cardiovascular disease, it is worth mentioning that two thirds of migraine patients have attacks without aura and that the absolute risk for cardiovascular disease is low in young women. Therefore, reassurance of these patients is important, given that four additional ischemic strokes per year in 10,000 women older than 45 years are attributable to migraine with aura [2, 51, 52].

However, it would be optimal to offer therapeutic options for a reduction of the increased cardiovascular risk in migraine patients. To reach this aim, knowledge on the pathogenesis of migraine, and, moreover, its associated cardiovascular complications, is essential. As described above, currently, vascular biomarkers have not yet unambiguously been identified, and it is not clear via which pathways the increased cardiovascular risk in migraine is generated. Nevertheless, it seems prudent to take additional cardiovascular risk factors (diabetes mellitus, arterial hypertension, and hyperlipidemia) into account, and smoking should be discouraged.

Further, recently the European Headache Federation (EHF) and the European Society of Contraception and Reproductive Health (ESC) have published a consensus statement concerning the prescription and usage of hormonal contraceptives in female migraineurs [21]. Specifically, the combination of smoking and oral contraceptives should be avoided in all cases in young women with migraine with aura, given the highly increased risk for ischemic stroke [34, 53]. Although an evidence-based approach for the prescription of oral contraceptives is lacking, clinicians are advised to take additional risk factors into account and to consider the type of hormonal contraception [21, 40]. Additional and comorbid risk factors for ischemic stroke, specifically in female migraineurs who use oral contraceptive medications, have been described as well, apart from the earlier cardiovascular risk factors. These include, for example, age older than 55 years, systemic diseases associated with stroke (sickle cell disorder and connective tissue disorder), cardiac disease with embolic potential, and previous history of deep vein thrombosis [21].

It is important to mention that the association between migraine and cerebrovascular disease is well documented in younger migraine patients, especially those with aura. However, prevalence estimates of vascular risk factors among elderly suffering from migraine without aura are lacking. Gilad et al. [54] designed a study to estimate the prevalence of vascular risk factors in the elderly population (older than 50 years old) with late onset of migraine without aura.

Advantages of the prescription of statins in the treatment of patients with migraine have been recommended by some authors, although their effectiveness has not been proven yet. Hypothesis concerning the site of action is that the anti-inflammatory properties of statins might influence the neurogenic inflammation [4]. However, statins might improve endothelial function, thus increasing the availability of NO and endothelium-dependent vasodilation—mechanisms involved in the pathophysiology of migraine, which might lead to worsening of migraine [55]. These disadvantageous speculations have not been clinically proven yet [4].

The antiplatelet drug aspirin has been mentioned in literature as a very effective first treatment for migraine attacks, mainly due to its analgesic properties [34]. However, *the Women's Health Study* has not proven any differences of the protective effects of aspirin on ischemic stroke in a female population with and without migraine. This encourages clinicians to weigh the advantages and disadvantages of aspirin usage, including higher bleeding risks. The study even mentions a potential harmful effect of aspirin in a small subgroup [56].

Lastly, evidences on the risk for stroke in triptan users are conflicting, but do not suggest strong cardiovascular safety issues. However, it is recommended to inform patients using ergot alkaloids about the risk of ischemic complications when ergot alkaloids are intensely consumed [57].

Taken together, as long as sound knowledge supporting a specific type of medication to reduce cardiovascular risk in migraine patients is not available yet, advise on a healthy lifestyle (mainly refraining from smoking and maintenance of a normal body weight) is a good first step [2, 5]. Nonetheless, migraine with aura should be regarded as an important risk factor—taking the patients' cardiovascular background into consideration as well [5].

2.7   Gaps and Future Research

Understanding the exact pathogenesis of migraine and the underlying biology of the link with cardiovascular disease is an important step. It is crucial to understand why migraine patients suffer from an increased systemic vascular malfunction (i.e., also in peripheral vessels outside the cranium) and whether this "vascular vulnerability" is causally related to the generation of migraine [5, 6].

Longitudinal studies assessing the factors involved in this relationship, also including specific subgroups who may be at higher risk, are needed. Factors such as the headache frequency and severity, as well as frequency of auras, should also be taken into account [2, 6].

Understanding the influence of (the combination of) the various risk factors could change our thinking of screening and recommended therapy, for example, by clarifying the role of age and gender. For example, these studies could examine whether migraine with aura should also be considered as a relevant risk factor for cardiovascular disease in male older migraineurs. Moreover, another relevant question might be whether the use of progesterone-only contraceptives (new-generation oral contraceptives) leads to an increased risk of stroke, as seems to be the case for combined hormonal contraceptives in patients with migraine with aura [21]. Enhancement of our understanding of the underlying biology could offer us answers to the question whether migraine is a modifiable vascular risk factor and whether precautions can be taken to reduce the increase in cardiovascular risk caused by migraine [5, 6].

Lastly, the establishment of specific and sensitive vascular biomarkers (e.g., [25]) would offer possibilities for early detection of vascular dysfunction in migraine patients and could, by identifying patients at risk, help to decrease future vascular events [6].

2.8   Conclusions

Although migraine is a highly prevalent disorder in the general population, its exact pathophysiological mechanisms have not been elucidated yet. The observed relation of migraine (with aura) with cardiovascular disease, mainly in women, raises more questions than it provides answers. Both might be expressions of a shared "vascular vulnerability." However, this correlation is complex and might be multifactorial, as several risk factors seem to have a more synergistic relationship. Pending specific knowledge on the mechanisms involved, therapies could focus mainly on an advanced life style, rather than a change in the patients' medication profile [51].

References

1. Sacco SCA. Migraine: an emerging cardiovascular risk factor. Cardiol Clin Pract. 2010;2(1):53–65.
2. Bigal ME, Kurth T, Hu H, Santanello N, Lipton RB. Migraine and cardiovascular disease: possible mechanisms of interaction. Neurology. 2009;72(21):1864–71.
3. Tepper D. Migraine and cardiovascular disease. Headache. 2014;54(7):1267–8.
4. Hu X, Zhou Y, Zhao H, Peng C. Migraine and the risk of stroke: an updated meta-analysis of prospective cohort studies. Neurol Sci. 2017;38(1):33–40.
5. Linstra KM, Ibrahimi K, Terwindt GM, Wermer MJ, MaassenVanDenBrink A. Migraine and cardiovascular disease in women. Maturitas. 2017;97:28–31.
6. Sacco S, Bushell C. Cardio-cerebrovascular comorbidity. In: Giamberardino MA, Martelletti P, editors. Comorbidities of headache disorders. New York, NY: Springer; 2017. p. 1–21.
7. Schurks M, Rist PM, Bigal ME, Buring JE, Lipton RB, Kurth T. Migraine and cardiovascular disease: systematic review and meta-analysis. BMJ. 2009;339:b3914.
8. Sacco S, Ornello R, Ripa P, Tiseo C, Degan D, Pistoia F, et al. Migraine and risk of ischaemic heart disease: a systematic review and meta-analysis of observational studies. Eur J Neurol. 2015;22(6):1001–11.
9. Kurth T, Winter AC, Eliassen AH, Dushkes R, Mukamal KJ, Rimm EB, et al. Migraine and risk of cardiovascular disease in women: prospective cohort study. BMJ. 2016;353: i2610.
10. Wang YC, Lin CW, Ho YT, Huang YP, Pan SL. Increased risk of ischemic heart disease in young patients with migraine: a population-based, propensity score-matched, longitudinal follow-up study. Int J Cardiol. 2014;172(1):213–6.
11. Bigal ME, Kurth T, Santanello N, Buse D, Golden W, Robbins M, et al. Migraine and cardiovascular disease: a population-based study. Neurology. 2010;74(8):628–35.
12. Gudmundsson LS, Scher AI, Aspelund T, Eliasson JH, Johannsson M, Thorgeirsson G, et al. Migraine with aura and risk of cardiovascular and all cause mortality in men and women: prospective cohort study. BMJ. 2010;341:c3966.
13. Kurth T, Gaziano JM, Cook NR, Bubes V, Logroscino G, Diener HC, et al. Migraine and risk of cardiovascular disease in men. Arch Intern Med. 2007;167(8):795–801.
14. Ahmed B, Bairey Merz CN, McClure C, Johnson BD, Reis SE, Bittner V, et al. Migraines, angiographic coronary artery disease and cardiovascular outcomes in women. Am J Med. 2006;119(8):670–5.
15. Velentgas P, Cole JA, Mo J, Sikes CR, Walker AM. Severe vascular events in migraine patients. Headache. 2004;44(7):642–51.
16. Hall GC, Brown MM, Mo J, MacRae KD. Triptans in migraine: the risks of stroke, cardiovascular disease, and death in practice. Neurology. 2004;62(4):563–8.
17. Sternfeld B, Stang P, Sidney S. Relationship of migraine headaches to experience of chest pain and subsequent risk for myocardial infarction. Neurology. 1995;45(12):2135–42.
18. Schwedt TJ. The migraine association with cardiac anomalies, cardiovascular disease, and stroke. Neurol Clin. 2009;27(2):513–23.
19. Alqaqa A. The Association of cardiovascular disease and migraine: review. J Clini Exp Cardiol. 2016;7(8):465.

20. Kruit MC, Van Buchem MA, Hofman PAM, Bakkers JTN, Terwindt GM, Ferrari MD, Launer LJ. Migraine as a risk factor for subclinical brain lesions. JAMA. 2004;291(4):427–34.

21. Sacco S, Merki-Feld GS, Ægidius KL, Bitzer J, Canonico M, Kurth T, et al. Hormonal contraceptives and risk of ischemic stroke in women with migraine: a consensus statement from the European Headache Federation (EHF) and the European Society of Contraception and Reproductive Health (ESC). J Headache Pain. 2017;18(1):108.

22. Bonetti PO, Lerman LO, Lerman A. Endothelial dysfunction: a marker of atherosclerotic risk. Arterioscler Thromb Vasc Biol. 2003;23(2):168–75.

23. Sacco S, Ripa P, Grassi D, Pistoia F, Ornello R, Carolei A, et al. Peripheral vascular dysfunction in migraine: a review. J Headache Pain. 2013;14:80.

24. Settakis G, Lengyel A, Molnár C, Bereczki D, Csiba L, Fülesdi B. Transcranial doppler study of the cerebral hemodynamic changes during breath-holding and hyperventilation tests. J Neuroimaging. 2002;12:252–8.

25. Ibrahimi K, De Graaf Y, Draijer R, Danser AHJ, Maassen VanDenBrink A, Van den Meiracker AH. Reproducibility and agreement of Different non-invasive methods of endothelial function assessment. Microvasc Res. 2018;117:50–6.

26. Butt JH, Franzmann U, Kruuse C. Endothelial function in migraine with aura - a systematic review. Headache. 2015;55(1):35–54.

27. Kernick D. Statins for all: should patients who have migraine with aura be on a statin? Br J Gen Pract. 2015;65(640):571–2.

28. Hanington E. Migraine: the platelet hypothesis after 10 years. Biomed Pharmacother. 1989;43(10):719–26.

29. Danese E, Montagnana M, Lippi G. Platelets and migraine. Thromb Res. 2014;134(1):17–22.

30. Govitrapong P, Limthavon C, Srikiatkhachorn A. 5-HT2 serotonin receptor on blood platelet of migraine patients. Headache. 1992;32(10):480–4.

31. Kozubski W, Walkowiak B, Cierniewski CS, Prusinski A. Platelet fibrinogen receptors in migraine patients. Headache. 1987;27(8):431–4.

32. Pawlowska Z, Kozubski W, Walkowiak B, Cierniewski CS. Increased platelet glycoprotein IIb reflects an abnormality of the platelet membrane in migraine. Headache. 1988;28(1):60.

33. Gupta VK. Patent foramen ovale closure and migraine: science and sensibility. Expert Rev Neurother. 2010;10(9):1409–22.

34. Silva IRFG. Migraine patients should be cautiously followed for risk factors leading to cardiovascular disease. Arq Neuropsiquiatr. 2013;71(2):119–24.

35. Dowson AJ, Wilmshurst P, Muir KW, et al. A prospective, multicentre, double-blind, placebo-controlled study to evaluate the efficacy of patent foramen ovale closure for the resolution of refractory migraine headache (the MIST Study): prevalence and size of shunts. Headache Care. 2005;2(4):223–7.

36. Colson NJ, Fernandez F, Lea RA, Griffiths LR. The search for migraine genes: an overview of current knowledge. Cell Mol Life Sci. 2007;64(3):331–44.

37. Gormley P, Anttila V, Winsvold BS, et al. Meta-analysis of 375,000 individuals identifies 38 susceptibility loci for migraine. Nat Genet. 2016;48(8):856–66.

38. Winsvold BS, Bettella F, Witoelar A, Anttila V, Gormley P, Kurth T, et al. Shared genetic risk between migraine and coronary artery disease: a genome-wide analysis of common variants. PLoS One. 2017;12(9):e0185663.

39. Weitzel KW, Strickland JM, Smith KM, Goode JV. Gender-specific issues in the treatment of migraine. J Gend Specif Med. 2001;4(1):64–74.

40. Sacco S, Ricci S, Degan D, Carolei A. Migraine in women: the role of hormones and their impact on vascular diseases. J Headache Pain. 2012;13(3):177–89.

41. Cook NR, Benseñor IM, Lotufo PA, Lee I, Skerrett PJ, Chown MJ, Ajani UA, Manson JE, Buring JE. Migraine and coronary heart disease in women and men. Headache. 2002;42:715–27.

42. Cook NR, Bensenor IM, Lotufo PA, Lee IM, Skerrett PJ, Chown MJ, et al. Migraine and coronary heart disease in women and men. Headache. 2002;42(8):715–27.

43. Chai NC, Peterlin BL, Calhoun AH. Migraine and estrogen. Curr Opin Neurol. 2014;27(3):315–24.
44. Gupta S, Mehrotra S, Villalon CM, Perusquia M, Saxena PR, MaassenVanDenBrink A. Potential role of female sex hormones in the pathophysiology of migraine. Pharmacol Ther. 2007;113(2):321–40.
45. Rosano GM, Leonardo F, Sarrel PM, Beale CM, De Luca F, Collins P. Cyclical variation in paroxysmal supraventricular tachycardia in women. Lancet. 1996;347(9004):786–8.
46. Lloyd GW, Patel NR, McGing E, Cooper AF, Brennand-Roper D, Jackson G. Does angina vary with the menstrual cycle in women with premenopausal coronary artery disease? Heart. 2000;84(2):189–92.
47. Choo WK. Menstruation angina: a case report. J Med Case Reports. 2009;3:6618.
48. Tietjen GE, Khubchandani J. Vascular biomarkers in migraine. Cephalalgia. 2015;35(2):95–117.
49. Tietjen GE, Khubchandani J, Herial N, Palm-Meinders IH, Koppen H, Terwindt GM, et al. Migraine and vascular disease biomarkers: a population-based case-control study. Cephalalgia. 2018;38:511.
50. Rose KM, Wong TY, Carson AP, Couper DJ, Klein R, Sharrett AR. Migraine and retinal microvascular abnormalities: the Atherosclerosis Risk in Communities Study. Neurology. 2007;68(20):1694–700.
51. Stam AH, Weller CM, Janssens ACJW, Aulchenko YS, Oostra BA, Frants RR, Van den Maagdenberg AMJM, Ferrari MD, Van Duijn CM, Terwindt GM. Migraine is not associated with enhanced atherosclerosis. Cephalalgia. 2013;33(4):228–35.
52. Kurth T, Diener HC. Migraine and stroke: perspectives for stroke physicians. Stroke. 2012;43(12):3421–6.
53. Chang CL, Donaghy M, Poulter N. Migraine and stroke in young women: case-control study. The World Health Organisation Collaborative Study of Cardiovascular Disease and Steroid Hormone Contraception. BMJ. 1999;318(7175):13–8.
54. Gilad R, Boaz M, Dabby R, Finkelstein V, Rapoport A, Lampl Y. Migraine and vascular risk factors in the elderly. Geriatr Gerontol Int. 2014;14(1):220–5.
55. John S, Schneider MP, Delles C, Jacobi J, Schmieder RE. Lipid-independent effects of statins on endothelial function and bioavailability of nitric oxide in hypercholesterolemic patients. Am Heart J. 2005;149(3):473.
56. Kurth T, Diener HC, Buring JE. Migraine and cardiovascular disease in women and the role of aspirin: subgroup analyses in the Women's Health Study. Cephalalgia. 2011;31(10):1106–15.
57. Roberto G, Raschi E, Piccinni C, Conti V, Vignatelli L, D'Alessandro R, et al. Adverse cardiovascular events associated with triptans and ergotamines for treatment of migraine: systematic review of observational studies. Cephalalgia. 2015;35(2):118–31.

Chapter 3
Sex- and Gender-Specific Aspects of Migraine Treatment

Daphne S. van Casteren, Emile G. M. Couturier, and Antoinette Maassen van den Brink

3.1 Gender Differences in Migraine Prevalence

The ratio of migraine prevalence between males and females varies throughout life. Overall, the prevalence of migraine is three times higher in females than in males. In young childhood the migraine prevalence is slightly higher in boys, while the prevalence is equal in prepubertal boys and girls. This balance turns into an increased migraine prevalence in girls after the age of menarche. Migraine peaks in prevalence in both sexes between 30 and 39 years of age [1–3]. During these fertile years, the menstruation is an important factor increasing the susceptibility for an upcoming attack [4]. Eventually, the difference in migraine prevalence between men and women becomes smaller in the postmenopausal period, but the prevalence remains slightly higher in women even after the age of 70 years [2, 3]. This course of gender differences in migraine prevalence throughout life suggests a prominent role for hormonal factors. It is important to mention that migraine is a multifactorial disease in which hormonal changes act as a triggering factor superimposed on a genetic predisposition.

D. S. van Casteren (✉)

Division of Pharmacology, Department of Internal Medicine, Erasmus Medical Center, Rotterdam, The Netherlands

Department of Neurology, Leiden University Medical Center, Leiden, The Netherlands
e-mail: d.s.van_casteren@lumc.nl

E. G. M. Couturier
Boerhaave Medisch Centrum, Amsterdam, The Netherlands

A. Maassen van den Brink
Division of Pharmacology, Department of Internal Medicine, Erasmus Medical Center, Rotterdam, The Netherlands
e-mail: a.vanharen-maassenvandenbrink@erasmusmc.nl

© Springer Nature Switzerland AG 2019
A. Maassen van den Brink, E. A. MacGregor (eds.), *Gender and Migraine*,
Headache, https://doi.org/10.1007/978-3-030-02988-3_3

3.2   Female-Specific Migraine Subtypes

Menstruation is an important factor increasing the susceptibility for an upcoming migraine attack, with the highest risk in the period of 2 days before the menstrual period until the first 3 days of bleeding (days −2 and +3 of the menstrual cycle) [4]. In general, these menstruation-associated migraine attacks are not preceded by an aura. In approximately 55% of female migraine patients, the attacks occur not only between days −2 and +3 but can also occur at other times of the menstrual cycle [5, 6]. According to the International Classification of Headache Disorders, 3rd edition, beta (ICHD-3 beta), this migraine subtype is called *menstrually related migraine without aura* [5]. A small proportion of female migraine patients, approximately 5.5%, experiences migraine attacks exclusively related to the menstruation [6]. This subtype is called *pure menstrual migraine without aura* [5]. Menstruation is considered to be endometrial bleeding resulting from either the normal menstrual cycle or from the withdrawal of exogenous progestogens, as in the use of combined oral contraceptives or cyclical hormone replacement therapy (HRT; oral or transdermal conjugated estrogens combined with cyclical oral progestogen). Headache or migraine that occurs for the first time in close temporal relation to regular use of exogenous hormones or pre-existing headache that significantly worsens after the start of such therapy is called *headache attributed to exogenous hormones*. It is reported in approximately 20–30% of women using exogenous hormones [7]. Discontinuation of exogenous estrogens, such as during the hormone-free interval of combined oral contraceptives, can induce headache or migraine. Typically, this *estrogen-withdrawal headache* occurs within 5 days after daily consumption of an exogenous estrogen for 3 weeks or longer, and it is reported in up to 70% of women using oral contraception [5, 8].

3.2.1   Migraine During Perimenopause and Postmenopause

Perimenopause describes the time when a woman's menstrual cycle changes from regular to irregular as a consequence of fluctuating ovarian activity. Menopause is defined as the day of the last menstruation. Perimenopause turns into postmenopause 12 months after the last menstruation [9]. Fluctuations in estrogen and progesterone levels during perimenopause are associated with increased susceptibility for migraine. This effect is seen on migraine attacks without aura, but not on migraine attacks with aura [9, 10]. After menopause, hormonal stability remains with high follicle-stimulating hormone (FSH) levels and low estrogen and progesterone levels due to decline of the production of these hormones by the ovaries. The postmenopausal status is associated with an improvement in migraine without aura. The frequency of migraine attacks decreases, and the attacks become less severe or even disappear [11–13]. Migraine prevalence in spontaneous menopausal women is 10.5%, which is considerably less than the 25% prevalence that is seen in premenopausal women. However, a migraine prevalence after a surgical menopause of 27% is approximately equal to the migraine prevalence in premenopausal women [13, 14]. In conclusion, migraine usually improves after spontaneous menopause, worsens during perimenopause, and remains the same after surgical menopause.

3.3   Hormonal Fluctuations Throughout the Menstrual Cycle

The median duration of a menstrual cycle is 28 days, and most cycle lengths are between 25 and 30 days. By definition, the first day of menstrual flow is called day +1, and there is no day 0. The menstrual cycle can be divided into two phases: (1) follicular or proliferative phase and (2) the luteal or secretory phase. The follicular phase starts on the first day of menstruation until ovulation. During this phase, the elevation of FSH causes follicles in the ovaries to grow. Ovulation, which is the release of a mature follicle, typically takes place at day 14 of the menstrual cycle and is caused by a sudden increase in luteinizing hormone (LH). This LH surge is initiated by an increase of estradiol produced by the preovulatory follicle and stimulates the synthesis of progesterone responsible for the midcycle FSH surge by luteinization of the granulosa cells. Ovulation is followed by the luteal phase. The remaining of an ovarian follicle that has released a mature oocyte during a previous ovulation is called the corpus luteum. It secretes a moderate amount of estrogen to inhibit further release of gonadotropin-releasing hormone (GnRH) and thus secretion of LH and FSH. The corpus luteum mainly secretes progesterone, which is responsible for the preparation of the uterine lining for pregnancy. If the corpus luteum is not rescued by pregnancy, progesterone withdrawal results in menses [15].

3.3.1   Role for Hormonal Fluctuations in Migraine

Clinical and epidemiological studies suggest a prominent role for sex hormones in female migraine patients. Onset of migraine increases at menarche, and after menopause the prevalence significantly declines [3]. As mentioned before, the menstruation and the menopausal transition phase are important factors increasing the susceptibility for migraine attacks. In contrast, pregnancy, lactation, and postmenopausal status are generally associated with an improvement in migraine [16]. Thus, sex hormonal conditions are known to affect the susceptibility for migraine attacks in women, but there is a lack of understanding of the exact underlying pathophysiological mechanism. Perimenstrual headache is commonly attributed to the sudden drop in estrogen prior to menses. A similar decrease in circulating estrogen occurs at ovulation, but this decline does not seem to be consistently related to increased provocation of migraine attacks [17, 18]. Therefore, increasing progesterone levels during ovulation may have migraine-preventive properties. In addition, the modest increase in migraine incidence around ovulation suggests that a sustained high level

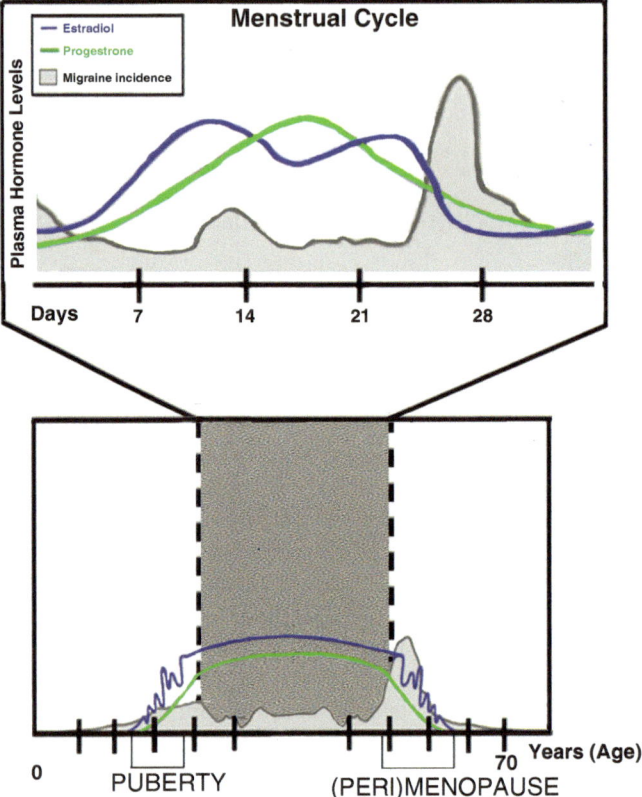

Fig. 3.1 Migraine incidence throughout a woman's life and hormonal fluctuations during the menstrual cycle

of estrogen is required before this drop in estrogen level in order to trigger an attack [19] (see Fig. 3.1).

3.3.2 Current Knowledge on Sex Hormone Levels in Women with Migraine

Results of studies regarding sex hormonal patterns in women with migraine are inconsistent. A recent study showed a faster decline in conjugated urinary estrogens in the late luteal phase compared to healthy controls (33.8 pg/mgCr; 95% CI, 28.0–40.8 vs. 23.1 pg/mgCr; 95% CI, 20.1–26.6; $p = 0.002$) without a significant difference in estrogen peak levels or mean daily levels between migraine patients and healthy controls [20]. Another study detected a significantly lower mean serum estradiol level on days 19–21 of the menstrual cycle of patients with MRM compared to healthy controls (mean ± SEM: 52 ± 4 pg/mL vs. 75 ± 8 pg/mL, $p = 0.014$), while no differences in estradiol levels were present at the onset of menstruation [21]. Both studies detected no significant differences in progesterone levels during the luteal phase or at the onset of menstruation. Mattsson found no statistical significant differences in serum levels of androstenedione, total testosterone, and free testosterone between postmenopausal migraine patients and healthy controls [22]. In addition, a study on salivary testosterone levels in chronic migraine patients, previously affected by medication-overuse headache, compared to healthy controls detected no significant differences between both groups (mean ± SEM: 47.74 ± 4.96 pg/mL in chronic migraineurs vs. 46.89 ± 4.17 pg/mL in controls) [23]. However, in a randomized clinical trial on the management of postmenopausal women with hormone therapy, a combination of 17β-estradiol and tibolone (a tissue-selective steroid with androgenic properties) was more effective in reducing the hours that migraine headache prohibited daily activities, compared to a combination of 17β-estradiol and estrogen-progesterone. These data suggest androgenic steroids might influence the clinical characteristics of migraine headache [24].

3.4 Female-Specific Migraine Treatments

Patients with PMM and MRM can be treated with acute and prophylactic drugs according to standard treatment strategy. There are no FDA-approved treatments specifically for this group of patients. However, multiple studies have shown the effectiveness of some non-specific and specific treatments in the acute and short-term preventive treatment of perimenstrual migraine attacks.

3.4.1 Acute Migraine Treatment Options in PMM and MRM

3.4.1.1 Acute Non-migraine-Specific Treatments

Menstrually related migraine attacks and non-menstrually related migraine attacks can be treated with non-specific analgesics (acetaminophen and NSAIDs) and anti-emetics. Perimenstrual attacks are generally more resistant to non-specific acute pharmacological treatment options compared to non-menstrual migraine attacks. However, a randomized controlled cross-over study with the objective to compare mefenamic acid (NSAID) with placebo in the acute treatment of menstrually related migraine attacks showed that mefenamic acid 500 mg three times daily had higher 2 h pain-free rates compared to placebo (66.6% vs. 8.3%; $p < 0.05$) [25]. Two replicate randomized placebo-controlled trials evaluated the efficacy of a naproxen 500 mg–sumatriptan 85 mg combination in the treatment of perimenstrual attacks. Naproxen–sumatriptan was statistically superior to placebo in both studies for 2 h and sustained headache-free responses [26].

3.4.1.2   Acute Migraine-Specific Treatments

Triptans and ergots are classes of migraine-specific acute treatments. An open-label study has been performed to assess the effectiveness of subcutaneous administration of dihydroergotamine in perimenstrual migraine attacks. Improvement in pain was seen in 83% of the participants. However, this result should be interpreted with caution because of a very low study quality [27]. Triptans are the treatment of choice for those attacks that do not respond adequately to non-specific analgesics. According to two systematic reviews on acute and prophylactic treatment options for menstrual migraine, almotriptan, sumatriptan, naratriptan, rizatriptan, and zolmitriptan have shown a statistically significant higher headache response after 2 and/or 4 h in triptan users compared to placebo [28, 29]. Controlled trials with the objective to compare frovatriptan to other triptans in the acute treatment of menstrually related migraine attacks have shown equal effectiveness in headache response after 2 h [30–32]. Recurrence rates of headache at 24 and 48 h were significantly lower with frovatriptan (17% and 21%) than with the comparators (27% and 31%; $p < 0.05$) in patients with oral contraceptive-induced menstrual migraine [30–32]. In conclusion, the efficacy at 2 h of triptans used for the acute treatment of migraine attacks has been shown to be similar during menstrual and non-menstrual periods, but the sustained response rates are lower during menstrual attacks [28, 33]. The higher headache recurrence rates may be the result of the persistence of the trigger (low estrogen levels and inflammation—prostaglandin synthesis) during menstruation [33]. Due to its sustained antimigraine effect, frovatriptan may be most suitable for the acute treatment of menstrually related migraine attacks.

3.4.2   Short-Term Prophylactic Treatment Options in PMM and MRM

3.4.2.1   Short-Term Non-migraine-Specific Treatments

Short-term or intermittent prophylaxis is the daily use of acute medication starting shortly before and during the menstrual period. The occurrence of perimenstrual migraine may be predictable in women with a regular menstrual cycle, allowing initiation of short-term prophylaxis a few days before the onset of an expected menstrual migraine attack. In general, short-lasting preventive medication is taken during 3–5 days before the onset of menstruation and continued during the first few days of bleeding. Naproxen and estrogens are described as non-migraine-specific pharmacological treatment options for this purpose. Naproxen 550 mg administered twice daily is the most commonly used NSAID for perimenstrual migraine prevention. However, this approach is based on a low level of evidence [34, 35]. Transdermal estradiol has been studied as short-term prophylactic treatment in patients with PMM and MRM. MacGregor et al. concluded estradiol 1.5 mg gel to be associated with a higher reduction in perimenstrual migraine days in the estradiol-treated cycles compared to placebo (RR 0.78; 95% CI 0.62–0.99; $p = 0.04$). However, estradiol treatment was followed by deferred estrogen withdrawal, triggering an increase in post-dosing migraine during the 5 days after the gel was stopped [36].

3.4.2.2 Short-Term Migraine-Specific Treatments

Information on the efficacy of ergots in short-term prophylaxis of perimenstrual migraine attacks is limited. A small open-label study investigated the effectiveness of a slow-release formulation of dihydroergotamine for this purpose. In the 16 patients who completed the study, both the intensity and duration of migraine significantly decreased during the treatment [37]. The highest-quality evidence for the use of triptans as short-term perimenstrual prevention exists for frovatriptan, for zolmitriptan, and to a lesser extent for naratriptan. Frovatriptan 2.5 mg both once and twice daily given prophylactically for 6 days, starting 2 days before the anticipated start of menstrually related migraine, appeared to be effective in reducing the incidence of menstrually related migraine, migraine severity, duration, and the use of rescue medication [38]. A second study was performed in patients with difficult to treat menstrually associated migraine, defined as having an inadequate response to at least one previous triptan. The mean number of headache-free perimenstrual periods significantly increased with frovatriptan treatment compared to placebo treatment [39]. In both studies a frovatriptan regimen of 2.5 mg twice a day was superior to a once-daily regimen. Tuchman et al. investigated the efficacy of zolmitriptan in short-term prevention of menstrually related migraine attacks and showed a higher >50% reduction in migraine attack frequency for both zolmitriptan 2.5 mg three times per day and zolmitriptan 2.5 mg twice per day compared to placebo (zolmitriptan three times daily 58.6%, $p = 0.0007$ vs. placebo; zolmitriptan twice daily 54.7%, $p = 0.002$ vs. placebo) [40]. Additionally, a comparative study between naratriptan 1 mg twice per day, naratriptan 2.5 mg twice per day, and placebo demonstrated a higher percentage of perimenstrual headache-free patients in the naratriptan 1 mg group compared to placebo (50% vs. 25%, $p = 0.003$), but not in the naratriptan 2.5 mg group [41]. Mannix et al. confirmed the efficacy of naratriptan 1 mg as short-term prevention measured by a significantly higher percentage of treated cycles without a menstrually associated migraine attack in naratriptan users compared to placebo [42]. In a systematic review, six trials involving frovatriptan, zolmitriptan, and naratriptan were reviewed as short-term prevention of menstrually related migraine attacks. Frovatriptan 2.5 mg twice per day and zolmitriptan 2.5 mg three times per day appeared to be the preferred regimens [43]. Only frovatriptan 2.5 mg twice per day received a level A rate of evidence and was determined to be effective for prevention of menstrually related migraine attacks according to the guidelines of the American Academy of Neurology and American Headache Society [44].

Importantly, when using triptans as short-term prophylaxis for menstrually associated migraine, the amount of medication used per month should not exceed the recommended maximum to prevent medication-overuse headache [45].

3.4.3   Female-Specific Prophylactic Treatment Options

3.4.3.1   Oral Contraceptives

Patients with PMM and MRM can be treated with prophylactic drugs according to standard treatment strategy. However, these prophylactics are often considered ineffective and frequently cause side effects. Clinical data on the preventive effect of combined oral contraceptives or progestogen-only contraceptives on PMM and MRM are scarce. Only a few open-label non-comparative studies are available in the literature, therefore diminishing the strength of the evidence. In addition, diagnoses are often inaccurate because no distinction is made between headache and migraine [7]. In general, after introducing a combined oral contraceptive, migraine can become worse (in approximately 25%), stay the same (in approximately 50%), or become less frequent (in approximately 25%) [7]. Different types and dosages of combined oral contraceptives do not have a significant influence on these results. The hormone-free interval of combined oral contraceptives can induce estrogen-withdrawal headache, which is reported in up to 70% of women using oral contraception [8]. Therefore, Sulak et al. and Coffee et al. investigated the effect of eliminating or shortening the hormone-free interval in combined oral contraceptive treatments. They concluded that compared to a 21/7 day regimen, a 168-day extended regimen resulted in a significant decrease in average daily headache score [17, 46]. However, extended use of combined oral contraceptives frequently results in breakthrough bleedings. Shortening, instead of eliminating, the hormone-free interval can minimize this risk of breakthrough bleedings. The efficacy of two combined oral contraceptive regimens (21 active pills + 7 placebo pills vs. 24 active pills + 4 placebo pills) has been compared in improving the severity of migraine attacks in patients with PMM. Both groups showed a significant reduction in intensity and duration of menstrual migraine attacks, but the 24/4 group reported a significantly greater reduction in intensity and duration compared to the 21/7 group [47].

The use of a daily progesterone-only pill inhibits ovulation and results in a stable estrogen production by the ovaries. Theoretically, the use of a progesterone-only pill could be effective as preventive treatment in migraine patients, especially in PMM and MRM. Two pilot studies on the effect of desogestrel 75 μg on migraine have been published. The first open-label observational study focused on the preventive effect of desogestrel 75 μg in migraine patients with aura. This study showed that 6 months of desogestrel use resulted in a significant reduction in migraine with aura attacks and in the duration of aura symptoms [48]. The second study is a small retrospective analysis of prospectively collected headache diaries. Merki-Feld et al. investigated the effectiveness of desogestrel 75 μg in women with migraine with aura and in women with migraine without aura as preventive migraine treatment. A significant reduction in migraine days (mean (SD) 5.2 (3.6) vs. 3.7 (3.4); $p = 0.001$), days with use of any pain medication (mean (SD) 5.7 (3.5) vs. 4.6 (2.5); $p = 0.007$), and headache intensity (mean (SD) 15.7 (10.4) vs. 10.4 (6.4); $p = 0.0001$) was observed after 3 months of desogestrel treatment [49]. The results of both studies should be interpreted cautiously because they were obtained in small study populations.

3.4.3.2   Other Female-Specific Prophylactic Migraine Treatments

Two nonrandomized open-label studies evaluated the effect of the GnRH agonist leuprolide acetate in treatment of severe or pharmacologically unresponsive menstrual migraine patients. Murray and Muse found in a small ($n = 5$) open-label trial significantly lower mean headache scores for the GnRH treatment months (3.75 mg IM, monthly) than for the control months [50]. Also Lichten et al. presented promising results concerning the preventive treatment with depo-leuprolide acetate 3.75 mg in patients with pharmacologically unresponsive MRM [51]. However, the results of these two studies should be interpreted with caution because of the open-label study design and small sample sizes. Additionally, notable adverse events were reported, especially hot flushes and severe daily migraine [50, 51]. Low-quality evidence have been obtained for the effect of magnesium, vitamin E, and phytoestrogens (estrogen-like molecules derived from soy) in the preventive treatment of menstrual migraine. The main limitations of the studies on these treatments are small sample sizes [52–55].

3.4.4   Migraine Treatment in Perimenopausal and Postmenopausal Women

Perimenopausal and postmenopausal migraine patients can be treated with acute and prophylactic drugs according to standard migraine treatments. Frequently, these patients continue suffering from disabling migraine attacks despite general migraine therapies [56]. Especially for these patients, the effect of various HRT strategies on migraine symptoms has been investigated. HRT is recommended for women with menopause before the age of 45 years to prevent long-term health consequences, including premature cardiovascular disease and sexual dysfunction. In addition, HRT is often prescribed to diminish perimenopausal complaints, such as vasomotor symptoms and sleep disturbances. Various cross-sectional studies found an association between migraine and current use of HRT. For instance, in postmenopausal women from the Women's Health Study, current HRT use was associated with a higher risk of migraine than nonuse (OR 1.42; 95% CI 1.24–1.62), both for users of estrogen plus progestin (OR 1.41; 95% CI 1.22–1.63) and users of estrogen alone (OR 1.39; 95% CI 1.14–1.69) [57]. The Norwegian Head-HUNT study showed also an association between migraine and current HRT use (OR 1.6; 95% CI 1.4–1.9) [58]. However, a questionnaire performed on perimenopausal and postmenopausal HRT users of the British Migraine Association showed a trend toward greater improvement of migraine in women using transdermal estrogen compared with oral conjugated estrogens [59]. In conclusion, due to inconsistent results, it is difficult to determine the effect of HRT on migraine during perimenopause and postmenopause.

3.5 Summary and Conclusion

The increased susceptibility for migraine attacks related to menstruation and the menopausal transition phase is most likely caused by hormonal fluctuations, but there is a lack of understanding of the exact underlying pathophysiological mechanism. Perimenstrual headache is commonly attributed to the sudden drop in estrogen prior to the menstruation. Recently, it was suggested that especially the rate of estrogen decline may be relevant for a difference between migraine patients and healthy controls. Additional research is needed to unravel the exact role of sex hormones in female migraine patients. The treatment of migraine triggered by hormonal changes is currently mainly based on consensus instead of real evidence. Despite the currently available treatments, especially in these migraine patients, high headache recurrence rates remain a problem. Hopefully, future research will lead to better treatment options with sustained efficacy.

References

1. Vetvik KG, MacGregor EA. Sex differences in the epidemiology, clinical features, and pathophysiology of migraine. Lancet Neurol. 2017;16(1):76–87.
2. Victor TW, Hu X, Campbell JC, Buse DC, Lipton RB. Migraine prevalence by age and sex in the United States: a life-span study. Cephalalgia. 2010;30(9):1065–72.
3. Stewart WF, Lipton RB, Celentano DD, Reed ML. Prevalence of migraine headache in the United States. Relation to age, income, race, and other sociodemographic factors. JAMA. 1992;267(1):64–9.
4. MacGregor EA, Hackshaw A. Prevalence of migraine on each day of the natural menstrual cycle. Neurology. 2004;63(2):351–3.
5. Headache Classification Committee of the International Headache Society (IHS). The International Classification of Headache Disorders, 3rd edition (beta version). Cephalalgia. 2013;33(9):629–808.
6. Pavlovic JM, Stewart WF, Bruce CA, Gorman JA, Sun H, Buse DC, et al. Burden of migraine related to menses: results from the AMPP study. J Headache Pain. 2015;16:24.
7. MacGregor EA. Contraception and headache. Headache. 2013;53(2):247–76.

8. Sulak PJ, Scow RD, Preece C, Riggs MW, Kuehl TJ. Hormone withdrawal symptoms in oral contraceptive users. Obstet Gynecol. 2000;95(2):261–6.
9. MacGregor EA. Migraine headache in perimenopausal and menopausal women. Curr Pain Headache Rep. 2009;13(5):399–403.
10. MacGregor EA. Perimenopausal migraine in women with vasomotor symptoms. Maturitas. 2012;71(1):79–82.
11. Silberstein SD, Merriam GR. Estrogens, progestins, and headache. Neurology. 1991;41(6):786–93.
12. Mattsson P. Hormonal factors in migraine: a population-based study of women aged 40 to 74 years. Headache. 2003;43(1):27–35.
13. Wang SJ, Fuh JL, Lu SR, Juang KD, Wang PH. Migraine prevalence during menopausal transition. Headache. 2003;43(5):470–8.
14. Lipton RB, Stewart WF, Diamond S, Diamond ML, Reed M. Prevalence and burden of migraine in the United States: data from the American Migraine Study II. Headache. 2001;41(7):646–57.
15. Reed BG, Carr BR. The normal menstrual cycle and the control of ovulation. In: De Groot LJ, Chrousos G, Dungan K, Feingold KR, Grossman A, Hershman JM, et al., editors. Endotext. South Dartmouth, MA: MDText.com, Inc.; 2000.
16. Macgregor EA. Headache in pregnancy. Continuum (Minneap Minn). 2014;20(1 Neurology of Pregnancy):128–47.
17. Sulak P, Willis S, Kuehl T, Coffee A, Clark J. Headaches and oral contraceptives: impact of eliminating the standard 7-day placebo interval. Headache. 2007;47(1):27–37.
18. Chai NC, Peterlin BL, Calhoun AH. Migraine and estrogen. Curr Opin Neurol. 2014;27(3):315–24.
19. Somerville BW. Estrogen-withdrawal migraine. I. Duration of exposure required and attempted prophylaxis by premenstrual estrogen administration. Neurology. 1975;25(3):239–44.
20. Pavlovic JM, Allshouse AA, Santoro NF, Crawford SL, Thurston RC, Neal-Perry GS, et al. Sex hormones in women with and without migraine: evidence of migraine-specific hormone profiles. Neurology. 2016;87(1):49–56.
21. Ibrahimi K, van Oosterhout WP, van Dorp W, Danser AH, Garrelds IM, Kushner SA, et al. Reduced trigeminovascular cyclicity in patients with menstrually related migraine. Neurology. 2015;84(2):125–31.
22. Mattsson P. Serum levels of androgens and migraine in postmenopausal women. Clin Sci (Lond). 2002;103(5):487–91.
23. Patacchioli FR, Monnazzi P, Simeoni S, De Filippis S, Salvatori E, Coloprisco G, et al. Salivary cortisol, dehydroepiandrosterone-sulphate (DHEA-S) and testosterone in women with chronic migraine. J Headache Pain. 2006;7(2):90–4.
24. Nappi RE, Sances G, Sommacal A, Detaddei S, Facchinetti F, Cristina S, et al. Different effects of tibolone and low-dose EPT in the management of postmenopausal women with primary headaches. Menopause (New York, NY). 2006;13(5):818–25.
25. Al-Waili NS. Treatment of menstrual migraine with prostaglandin synthesis inhibitor mefenamic acid: double-blind study with placebo. Eur J Med Res. 2000;5(4):176–82.
26. Mannix LK, Martin VT, Cady RK, Diamond ML, Lener SE, White JD, et al. Combination treatment for menstrual migraine and dysmenorrhea using sumatriptan-naproxen: two randomized controlled trials. Obstet Gynecol. 2009;114(1):106–13.
27. Diamond S, Freitag FG, Diamond ML, Urban GJ. Subcutaneous dihydroergotamine mesylate (DHE) in the treatment of menstrual migraine. Headache Quart. 1996;7(2):145–7.
28. Maasumi K, Tepper SJ, Kriegler JS. Menstrual migraine and treatment options: review. Headache. 2017;57(2):194–208.
29. Nierenburg Hdel C, Ailani J, Malloy M, Siavoshi S, Hu NN, Yusuf N. Systematic review of preventive and acute treatment of menstrual migraine. Headache. 2015;55(8):1052–71.
30. Savi L, Omboni S, Lisotto C, Zanchin G, Ferrari MD, Zava D, et al. Efficacy of frovatriptan in the acute treatment of menstrually related migraine: analysis of a double-blind, randomized, cross-over, multicenter, Italian, comparative study versus rizatriptan. J Headache Pain. 2011;12(6):609–15.

31. Savi L, Omboni S, Lisotto C, Zanchin G, Ferrari MD, Zava D, et al. A double-blind, randomized, multicenter, Italian study of frovatriptan versus rizatriptan for the acute treatment of migraine. J Headache Pain. 2011;12(2):219–26.
32. Allais G, Tullo V, Omboni S, Pezzola D, Zava D, Benedetto C, et al. Frovatriptan vs. other triptans for the acute treatment of oral contraceptive-induced menstrual migraine: pooled analysis of three double-blind, randomized, crossover, multicenter studies. Neurol Sci. 2013;34(Suppl 1):S83–6.
33. Pringsheim T, Davenport WJ, Dodick D. Acute treatment and prevention of menstrually related migraine headache: evidence-based review. Neurology. 2008;70(17):1555–63.
34. Sances G, Martignoni E, Fioroni L, Blandini F, Facchinetti F, Nappi G. Naproxen sodium in menstrual migraine prophylaxis: a double-blind placebo controlled study. Headache. 1990;30(11):705–9.
35. Allais G, Bussone G, De Lorenzo C, Castagnoli Gabellari I, Zonca M, Mana O, et al. Naproxen sodium in short-term prophylaxis of pure menstrual migraine: pathophysiological and clinical considerations. Neurol Sci. 2007;28(Suppl 2):S225–8.
36. MacGregor EA, Frith A, Ellis J, Aspinall L, Hackshaw A. Prevention of menstrual attacks of migraine: a double-blind placebo-controlled crossover study. Neurology. 2006;67(12):2159–63.
37. D'Alessandro R, Gamberini G, Lozito A, Sacquegna T. Menstrual migraine: intermittent prophylaxis with a timed-release pharmacological formulation of dihydroergotamine. Cephalalgia. 1983;3(Suppl 1):156–8.
38. Silberstein SD, Elkind AH, Schreiber C, Keywood C. A randomized trial of frovatriptan for the intermittent prevention of menstrual migraine. Neurology. 2004;63(2):261–9.
39. Brandes JL, Poole A, Kallela M, Schreiber CP, MacGregor EA, Silberstein SD, et al. Short-term frovatriptan for the prevention of difficult-to-treat menstrual migraine attacks. Cephalalgia. 2009;29(11):1133–48.
40. Tuchman MM, Hee A, Emeribe U, Silberstein S. Oral zolmitriptan in the short-term prevention of menstrual migraine: a randomized, placebo-controlled study. CNS Drugs. 2008;22(10):877–86.
41. Newman L, Mannix LK, Landy S, Silberstein S, Lipton RB, Putnam DG, et al. Naratriptan as short-term prophylaxis of menstrually associated migraine: a randomized, double-blind, placebo-controlled study. Headache. 2001;41(3):248–56.
42. Mannix LK, Savani N, Landy S, Valade D, Shackelford S, Ames MH, et al. Efficacy and tolerability of naratriptan for short-term prevention of menstrually related migraine: data from two randomized, double-blind, placebo-controlled studies. Headache. 2007;47(7):1037–49.
43. Hu Y, Guan X, Fan L, Jin L. Triptans in prevention of menstrual migraine: a systematic review with meta-analysis. J Headache Pain. 2013;14:7.
44. Silberstein SD, Holland S, Freitag F, Dodick DW, Argoff C, Ashman E. Evidence-based guideline update: pharmacologic treatment for episodic migraine prevention in adults: report of the Quality Standards Subcommittee of the American Academy of Neurology and the American Headache Society. Neurology. 2012;78(17):1337–45.
45. Tepper SJ. Medication-overuse headache. Continuum (Minneap Minn). 2012;18(4):807–22.
46. Coffee AL, Sulak PJ, Hill AJ, Hansen DJ, Kuehl TJ, Clark JW. Extended cycle combined oral contraceptives and prophylactic frovatriptan during the hormone-free interval in women with menstrual-related migraines. J Womens Health (Larchmt). 2014;23(4):310–7.
47. De Leo V, Scolaro V, Musacchio MC, Di Sabatino A, Morgante G, Cianci A. Combined oral contraceptives in women with menstrual migraine without aura. Fertil Steril. 2011;96(4):917–20.
48. Nappi RE, Sances G, Allais G, Terreno E, Benedetto C, Vaccaro V, et al. Effects of an estrogen-free, desogestrel-containing oral contraceptive in women with migraine with aura: a prospective diary-based pilot study. Contraception. 2011;83(3):223–8.
49. Merki-Feld GS, Imthurn B, Langner R, Sandor PS, Gantenbein AR. Headache frequency and intensity in female migraineurs using desogestrel-only contraception: a retrospective pilot diary study. Cephalalgia. 2013;33(5):340–6.
50. Murray SC, Muse KN. Effective treatment of severe menstrual migraine headaches with gonadotropin-releasing hormone agonist and "add-back" therapy. Fertil Steril. 1997;67(2):390–3.

51. Lichten EM, Lichten JB, Whitty AJ, Pieper D. The use of leuprolide acetate in the diagnosis and treatment of menstrual migraine: the role of artifically-induced menopause. Headache Quart. 1995;6(4):313–6.
52. Ziaei S, Kazemnejad A, Sedighi A. The effect of vitamin E on the treatment of menstrual migraine. Med Sci Monit. 2009;15(1):Cr16–9.
53. Ferrante F, Fusco E, Calabresi P, Cupini LM. Phyto-oestrogens in the prophylaxis of menstrual migraine. Clin Neuropharmacol. 2004;27(3):137–40.
54. Burke BE, Olson RD, Cusack BJ. Randomized, controlled trial of phytoestrogen in the prophylactic treatment of menstrual migraine. Biomed Pharmacother. 2002;56(6):283–8.
55. Facchinetti F, Sances G, Borella P, Genazzani AR, Nappi G. Magnesium prophylaxis of menstrual migraine: effects on intracellular magnesium. Headache. 1991;31(5):298–301.
56. Martin VT, Pavlovic J, Fanning KM, Buse DC, Reed ML, Lipton RB. Perimenopause and menopause are associated with high frequency headache in women with migraine: results of the American migraine prevalence and prevention study. Headache. 2016;56(2):292–305.
57. Misakian AL, Langer RD, Bensenor IM, Cook NR, Manson JE, Buring JE, et al. Postmenopausal hormone therapy and migraine headache. J Womens Health (Larchmt). 2003;12(10):1027–36.
58. Aegidius KL, Zwart JA, Hagen K, Schei B, Stovner LJ. Hormone replacement therapy and headache prevalence in postmenopausal women. The Head-HUNT study. Eur J Neurol. 2007;14(1):73–8.
59. MacGregor A. Effects of oral and transdermal estrogen replacement on migraine. Cephalalgia. 1999;19(2):124–5.

Chapter 4
Headache and Pregnancy

Andrea Negro and Dimos Dimitrios Mitsikostas

4.1 Introduction

Headache is the most frequent neurologic disorder observed in the outpatient setting. The Global Burden of Disease (GBD) ranked headache disorders as the seventh cause of years lived with disability (YLDs) [1].

The first step when approaching headache is to distinguish a primary headache from a secondary headache, when pain is not the disease but a symptom of another disorder. This differential diagnosis is even more important during pregnancy.

There are three possible scenarios for a pregnant woman suffering from headache [2, 3]:

1. The occurrence of her usual headache
2. The occurrence for the first time in her life of severe headache
3. The occurrence of pain that is different in quality, intensity, or associated symptoms from her usual primary headache

In the last two scenarios, an appropriate diagnostic evaluation is mandatory because headache could be a symptom of an underlying disease.

A. Negro (✉)
Department of Clinical and Molecular Medicine, Regional Referral Headache Centre,
Sant'Andrea Hospital, Sapienza University of Rome, Rome, Italy
e-mail: andrea.negro@uniroma1.it

D. D. Mitsikostas
Neurology Department, Aeginition Hospital, National and Kapodistrian University of Athens,
Athens, Greece

© Springer Nature Switzerland AG 2019
A. Maassen van den Brink, E. A. MacGregor (eds.), *Gender and Migraine*,
Headache, https://doi.org/10.1007/978-3-030-02988-3_4

4.2 Clinical Headache Phenotypes and Observational Studies in Pregnancy

4.2.1 Primary Headaches

Migraine and tension-type headache (TTH) are the more frequent conditions affecting women asking medical consultation. Hormonal changes influence the course of primary headaches during pregnancy (Table 4.1), sometimes with a change in pattern from migraine without aura (MO) to migraine with aura (MA) and vice versa or from MO to TTH and vice versa.

4.2.1.1 Migraine

About 50–75% of women experience a significant improvement in migraine during pregnancy with a marked reduction in intensity and frequency of attacks and sometimes also a complete resolution (Table 4.1) [4–13]. The improvement occurs

Table 4.1 Primary headaches course during pregnancy (Modified from [28])

Author	Study design	Sample size (*n*)	Population charactheristics	Improvement or remission (%)	Unchanged (%)	Worsening (%)
Migraine without aura						
Granella et al. [4]	R	571	Full sample size, 1300 women; 943 had had pregnancies; 571 women with migraine before first pregnancy	67.3	29.2	3.5
Scharff et al. [5]	P	19	Full sample size, 30; 11/30 with headache onset during pregnancy	56.7	36.6	6.7
Maggioni et al. [6]	R	81	Full sample size, 430 women, interviewed 3 days after delivery; among them, 81 MO, 12 MA, 33 TTH	89.5	7.7	2.5
Marcus et al. [7]	P	49	16 M, 16 TTH, 15 M + TTH. Headache recorded daily during pregnancy and 3 months postpartum	40.8	51	8.2
Granella et al. [8]	R	200	100 MA and 200 MO as controls	76.8	22.2	1
Sances et al. [9]	P	47	Full sample size, 49; 2 MA, 47 MO	87.2	12.8	0
Mattsson [10]	R	728	Full sample size, 728; full information available for 102 women	81.4	17.6	1

Table 4.1 (continued)

Author	Study design	Sample size (n)	Population charactheristics	Improvement or remission (%)	Unchanged (%)	Worsening (%)
Kelman [11]	R	504	Greater improvement in MO patients rather than MA patients	38.2	27.8	34
Ertesvåg et al. [12]	P	410	Full sample size, 1361 women. 410 with M	65.9	19.8	14.4
Melhado et al. [13]	P	737	Full sample size, 1101 women. 737 with M. Data partially derived from graphics	65	26.1	8.9
Summary		3346		66.9	25.8	8
Migraine with aura						
Maggioni et al. [6]	R	12	430 women 3 days after delivery; among them, 81 MO, 12 MA, 33 TTH	83.4	16.6	0
Granella et al. [8]	R	100	100 MA and 200 MO as controls	43.6	48.7	7.7
Mattsson [10]	R	728	Full sample size, 728; full information available for 23 women	78.3	4.3	17.4
Summary		840		68.4	23.2	8.4
Tension-type headache						
Maggioni et al. [6]	R	33	Full sample size, 430 women, interviewed 3 days after delivery; among them, 81 MO, 12 MA, 33 TTH	82.1	17.9	0
Melhado et al. [13]	P	112	Full sample size, 1101 women. 112 with TTH. Data derived from graphics	N/A (≈60)	N/A (≈35)	N/A (≈5)
Summary		145		–	–	–
Cluster headache						
van Vliet et al. [23]	R	53	Full sample size, 196 CH; 53 had their first attack before the first pregnancy. 23% of episodic CH patients reported that an "expected" cluster period did not occur during pregnancy. Here improvement includes eight patients who had a cluster period within 1 month after delivery.	69.9	20.7	9.4

P prospective, *R* retrospective, *M* migraine, *MO* migraine without aura, *MA* migraine with aura, *TTH* tension-type headache, *CH* cluster headache during the first trimester, with a further reduction during the second and third ones [5, 6, 9]. Consequently, the 1-year headache prevalence of migraine is lower among nulliparous pregnant women than in nonpregnant women [14].

A large Italian study found that the onset of migraine at menarche and menstrual migraine correlated with a significantly higher percentage of remissions during pregnancy [8], but the following studies did not confirm this data [7, 9, 11].

Usually, none of the women experiencing a complete remission during the first two trimesters shows a recurrence of migraine attacks before delivery [9], even if a study showed a U-shaped curve in migraine evolution during pregnancy in multiparous women with an increase in headache burden already in the 4 weeks before birth [5].

A mean of 25% of MO patients do not improve during pregnancy, with pregestation menstrual-related migraine, hyperemesis, and pathological pregnancy course being linked with the persistence of the attacks (Table 4.1) [9, 15].

Migraine can also worsen during pregnancy, particularly in the first trimester, as reported by 8% of women (Table 4.1) [4–13].

Pluripara mothers are more likely to experience worsening of headache [5]. This is in line with the evidence that half of the multiparous subjects present a persistent worsening of their headache with following gestations [6].

In the particular case of in vitro fertilization and embryo-transfer treatments, the prevalence of headache attacks is higher at the first stage of the procedure (due to GnRH analogue administration) and at the end of the protocol in case there is no conception [16]; that happens because in both the situations there is a decline in blood estrogen levels.

Only few studies evaluated the clinical course of MA during pregnancy (Table 4.1). MA starts during pregnancy more frequently than MO does (in 10.7 up to 14% vs. 1 up to 10% of case, respectively) [6, 8, 12, 13, 17]. The majority of patients improve during pregnancy, but worsening occurs in 8.4% of MA women.

Gestation may trigger attacks of aura without headache [18], as MA can develop new aura symptoms during gestation as well [19, 20].

Postpartum headache occurs in about 30–40% of all women, not only in those with migraine [5, 9]. A large prospective trial found an increase in headache intensity, pain duration, and analgesic therapies during puerperium [16].

Most of the attacks develop during the first week after delivery, with headache during pregnancy and regional anesthesia injections as risk factors [21].

Breastfeeding and age >30 years may retard headache recurrence, but in half of women, prepregnancy headache pattern restores within 1 month from delivery [9]. The rapid return of migraine attacks can be explained by the abrupt fall in estrogen levels, by the implications of the new parental role (anxiety, worry, and sleep deprivation), and also by a postpartum depression.

4.2.1.2   Tension-Type Headache

TTH accounts for the 26% of headaches during pregnancy [22]. A study found significantly higher remission and improvement rates than in MO (Table 4.1) [6]. This evidence is explained by the fact that female hormones modulate serotonin and endorphins, which are involved in TTH pathophysiology [3]. TTH worsens in 5% of cases during gestation [13], and, according to some authors, it never does [6].

4.2.1.3 Cluster Headache

Cluster headache (CH) is seen in less than 0.3% of pregnancies [22]. The onset of first attacks during pregnancy is rare. Usually intensity and frequency of CH attacks do not change in the majority of cases, but nearly 25% of pregnant women report that an expected cluster period does not occur during gestation while it may develop soon after delivery [23].

The prospective of the treatment limitations in case of CH during pregnancy explains why women having the onset of CH before their first pregnancy usually have fewer children than those women who were already mothers at the time of the first attack [23].

4.2.2 Secondary Headaches

Pregnancy is a known risk factor for a secondary headache disorder. Among pregnant women presenting with acute headache, the percentage of secondary forms ranges from 14.3% to 52.6% [13, 24, 25]. Hypertensive disorders of pregnancy covered half of these cases, with preeclampsia as the major cause [24].

Hormonal changes, hypercoagulability, and anesthesia for labor are just some of the many factors contributing to the high incidence of secondary headaches during gestation.

Among patients with a primary headache history, any change in pattern of previous headache as longer attack duration is the most common feature suggesting a secondary headache [24, 25]. Secondary and primary headache features may not differ, making the differential diagnosis a true challenge, even more if considering that migraine is per se an independent risk factor for the development of secondary headaches [26].

It is fundamental looking for the well-known red flags suggesting for a secondary origin of an acute headache during pregnancy (Table 4.2) [24]. Between them, lack of headache history, abnormalities at neurologic examination, and elevated blood pressure are those of primary importance. The presence of one of those red flags makes brain MRI or CT scans often mandatory [27].

The main conditions associated with secondary headache are preeclampsia, cerebral venous thrombosis (CVT), ischemic or hemorrhagic stroke, subarachnoid hemorrhage (SAH), arterial dissection, reversible cerebral vasoconstriction syndrome (RCVS), posterior reversible leukoencephalopathy syndrome (PRES), idiopathic intracranial hypertension (IIH), and pituitary apoplexy (Table 4.3) [28].

Table 4.2 Red Flags for headache in pregnancy (Modified from [28])

1. Headache that peaks in severity in less than 5 min (thunderclap headache)
2. New onset headache or change in pattern of previous headache
3. Headache changing with posture (e.g., standing up)
4. Headache awakening the pregnant
5. Headache precipitated by physical activity or Valsalva maneuver (e.g., coughing, laughing, straining)
6. Side-locked headache
7. Thrombophilia
8. Neurological symptoms or signs
9. Head/neck injury or trauma
10. Fever
11. Seizures
12. Elevated blood pressure
13. Systemic illness, weight loss
14. History of malignancy
15. History of HIV or active infections
16. History of pituitary disorders
17. Recent travel at risk of infective disease

Modified from Mitsikostas et al. [37] (European Headache Federation consensus on technical investigation for primary headache disorders)

Table 4.3 Main causes of secondary headache in pregnant women

Secondary headaches during pregnancy	
Arterial dissection	Intracranial hypotension
Arteriovenous malformation	Ischemic stroke
Brain tumors	Meningitis/encephalitis
Cerebral venous thrombosis (CVT)	Pituitary adenoma
Choriocarcinoma	Pituitary apoplexy
Cranial neuralgias	Pituitary meningioma
Dehydration	Reversible posterior leukoencephalopathy syndrome (PRES)
Eclampsia and preeclampsia	Reversible vasoconstriction syndrome (RCVS)
Head trauma	Sinusitis
Idiopathic intracranial hypertension (IIH)	Subarachnoid hemorrhage (SAH)
Intracranial hemorrhage (ICH)	Vasculitis

4.2.2.1 Preeclampsia and Eclampsia

Preeclampsia is a complication present in 5% of pregnancies [29]. The typical presentation of this condition is a progressive bilateral pulsating headache that occurs in pregnancy or in the puerperium. The headache can be associated with visual changes similar to the typical visual aura and is often aggravated by physical activity. It is poorly responsive to over-the-counter drugs but resolves within a week after blood pressure adjustment [3]. According to the International Classification of Headache Disorders (ICHD-3beta), at least two of the following three characteristics are required for the diagnosis: (a) bilateral location, (b) pulsating quality, and (c) aggravated by physical activity [30].

4.2.2.2 Cerebral Venous Thrombosis

Headache occurs in 80–90% of cases of CVT but lacks specific characteristics: more frequently it is progressive, diffuse, and severe, but it can also be sudden (even thunderclap), unilateral, and mild [31]. The headache in CVT is often associated with focal signs (seizures or neurological deficits) and/or signs of intracranial hypertension (nausea and papilledema), cavernous sinus syndrome, or subacute encephalopathy, with a mortality rate of up to 30% [22].

4.2.2.3 Ischemic Stroke

Headache is present in up to one-third ischemic stroke especially in those within the posterior circulation. It can be unilateral, ipsilateral, or bilateral to the stroke. Headache has no specific characteristics, and it is usually of moderate intensity with a self-limited course [32].

Rarely, an acute ischemic stroke can present with an isolated sudden (even thunderclap) headache, but most frequently focal signs and/or alterations of consciousness overshadow the headache [33]. The diagnosis and the causal link with ischemic stroke are easy, because the headache occurs both acutely and with neurological signs and because it often remits rapidly. The differential diagnosis with primary headaches is facilitated by the neurological signs, but it is important to remember that migraine is per se an independent risk factor ischemic stroke [26].

4.2.2.4 Subarachnoid Hemorrhage

SAH is a severe condition with a mortality rate of 40–50%, and because of its rapid progression 10–20% of patients die before arriving at hospital. SAH presents a 20-fold increased risk in the puerperium, and a thunderclap headache is usually the prominent symptom [22].

The pain is severe and sudden, typically peaking in seconds or minutes, and often followed by vomiting and loss of consciousness [34].

The abrupt onset helps to distinguish the headache associated to SAH from primary headaches with thunderclap features (e.g., associated with sexual activity or exercise).

4.2.2.5 Arterial Dissection

Cervical carotid, vertebral, and intracranial artery dissections are rare complications of pregnancy and puerperium. Arterial dissections are usually associated with pre-eclampsia [35]. Headache is most frequently the first symptom. Pain is severe, sudden (even thunderclap), and unilateral (ipsilateral to the dissected vessel). Headache persists for days and can be a warning symptom preceding ischemic infarcts.

4.2.2.6 Reversible Cerebral Vasoconstriction Syndrome

RCVS usually occurs in the postpartum period within a week after delivery. The condition can be associated with fluctuating focal neurological deficits and seizures, but a thunderclap headache is often the only symptom. The pain is severe and diffuse, often triggered by exertion, sexual activity, Valsalva maneuvers, and/or emotion [36]. Headache usually relapses within a few days, recurring over 1–2 weeks, and resolving by 12 weeks after clinical onset [15, 37].

4.2.2.7 Posterior Reversible Encephalopathy Syndrome

PRES is a neuroradiological clinical entity more common in women and unusual after delivery. It is often associated with preeclampsia, eclampsia, renal failure, hypertensive encephalopathy, RCVS, immunosuppressive therapy, or chemotherapy [38]. The most common symptom is headache, usually described as occipital and bilateral and dull in nature, in association with impaired consciousness, seizures, focal neurological signs, visual changes or blindness, nausea, and vomiting. Symptoms occur without prodrome, progress over 12–48 h, and generally resolve within a period of days or weeks when prompt diagnosis is established and appropriate treatment is started without delay [39]. On the contrary recovery of the MRI abnormalities takes longer.

4.2.2.8 Idiopathic Intracranial Hypertension

IIH usually occurs during the first trimester in obese women. It is characterized by severe visual deficits, papilledema, tinnitus, or sixth nerve palsies [22, 37, 40]. Patients can suffer from a progressive, daily headache, frequently described as frontal, retro-orbital, "pressure-like," or explosive. Headache is typically aggravated by Valsalva maneuvers and position change. Migraine-like headache may also occur.

4.2.2.9 Pituitary Apoplexy

Pituitary apoplexy is a rare, acute, and life-threatening condition [41]. A severe and sudden headache is the most frequent presentation of rapid enlargement of non-functioning pituitary macroadenomas resulting from hemorrhage and/or infarction.

Differential diagnosis is with other causes of thunderclap headache [42]. Pituitary apoplexy should be suspected in case of a sudden and severe headache associated with ophthalmoplegia, nausea, vomiting, altered consciousness, visual symptoms, and hypopituitarism [3, 40].

4.3 Treatment of Headaches in Pregnancy and Breastfeeding Women

During pregnancy and breastfeeding, an under-management of headache can have negative effects for both the mother and the newborn as consequence of stress, depression, sleep deprivation, and poor nutritional intake. Nevertheless, the preferred therapeutic strategy should always be a non-pharmacological one. Most patients are not aware that inadvertent exposure to teratogenic agents can lead to irreversible fetal malformations [37].

If non-pharmacological interventions seem inadequate, the basic rule is to choose the lowest effective dose for the shortest duration of treatment, taking always into account all the benefits and possible risks of a given medication (Table 4.4).

Table 4.4 Summarizing table on treatment of headache in pregnant and breastfeeding women

Medication	Adverse effects	Comments
Pregnancy		
Paracetamol	–	Preferred acute treatment
Aspirin (ASA)	>100 mg/day or TR3: premature closure of ductus arteriosus, oligohydramnios, neonatal bleeding	– <100 mg/day seems safe – Caution in TR1 and TR2 – Avoid in TR3
Caffeine	–	–
NSAIDs (nonselective): Ibuprofen, naproxen, diclofenac, indomethacin	– TR1: miscarriage – TR3: premature closure ductus arteriosus, impaired renal function, cerebral palsy, intraventricular hemorrhage	– Can be used safely during TR2 – Avoid in TR3 – Selective COX inhibitors contraindicated
Triptans: Sumatriptan, zolmitriptan, eletriptan, rizatriptan	No major congenital defects	Appropriate if benefit outweighs risk
Oxygen	–	Preferred acute treatment in CH
Lidocaine	–	– Second-line acute treatment in CH – Intranasal formulation preferred
Corticosteroids: Prednisone, prednisolone	–	– Avoid during first semester – Low doses recommended – Reserved for CH or status migrainosus

(continued)

Table 4.4 (continued)

Medication	Adverse effects	Comments
Opioids: Tramadol, codeine	– MOH – Withdrawal symptoms and respiratory depression in the newborn	– Not considered first-line treatment in primary headaches – Caution in TR1 and TR2 – Avoid in TR3
Ergots/ergots alkaloids	– Uterotonic and vasoconstrictive effect – Fetal distress – CM	Avoid in any trimester
β-blockers: Metoprolol, propranolol	Neonatal bradycardia, hypotension, hypoglycemia when exposed in TR3	– First-line migraine prophylaxis – If possible taper off TR3 – Monitor newborn exposed in TR3
ACE-I, ARB	CM	Avoid in any trimester
Verapamil	–	First-line CH profylaxis
TCA	–	– Second-line migraine prophyaxis when β-blocker ineffective/contraindicated – Amytriptiline preferred
Venlafaxine	CM	Should be avoided
Duloxetine	–	No reported AE
Valproate	Neural tube defects, cardiac defects, urinary tract defects, cleft palate, lower IQ scores	Avoid in any trimester
Topiramate	Cleft lip/palate, low birth weight	Avoid in any trimester
Gabapentin	–	Limited data
Lamotrigine	No major congenital defects	Safest antiepileptic drug
Flunarizine	–	Not recommended (no data available)
Lithium	– Congenital cardiac malformations and cardiac arrhythmias – Anomalies of the CNS and endocrine system – Polyhydramnios – Stillbirth	Not recommended but can be considered in uncontrolled CH refractory to verapamil
Botulinum toxin A	–	No reported AE when injected correctly
Nerve blocks	–	– No reported AE when injected correctly – Preferred agent: lidocaine
Magnesium	– High-dose I.V.: bone abnormalities – Possible transient neurological symptoms and hypotonia after delivery	– Appropriate in any trimester; caution directly before delivery – Chronic use of oral magnesium: controversial
Coenzyme Q10	–	No reported AE
Butterbur, feverfew, high-dosed riboflavine	–	Not recommended

Table 4.4 (continued)

Medication	Adverse effects	Comments
Breastfeeding		
Paracetamol	–	Preferred acute treatment
Aspirin (ASA)	Reye's syndrome	Not recommended
Caffeine	–	Moderate dosage
NSAIDs (Nonselective): Ibuprofen, naproxen, indomethacin	Aggravation of jaundice	Ibuprofen preferred
Triptans	–	– Sumatriptan: no need to "pump and dump" – Less evidence on the other triptans: avoid nursing for 24 h after use of triptan as extra safety measurement
Oxygen	–	Preferred acute treatment in CH
Lidocaine	–	– Second-line acute treatment in CH – Intranasal formulation preferred
Corticosteroids: Prednisone, prednisolone	Prolonged high-dosed therapy: infant growth and development can be affected	Intravenously: delay breastfeeding for 2–8 h
Opioids: Tramadol, codeine	Sedation and respiratory depression in the infant	Not considered first-line treatment in primary headaches
Ergots/ergots alkaloids	– Vomiting, diarrhea, convulsions – Decrease of prolactine in the mother	Avoid in any trimester
β-blockers: Metoprolol, propranolol	– Hypotension, bradycardia – Weakness	– Metoprolol preferred – Avoid in children with astma
ACE-I, ARB	Impact on kidney development	Probably compatible (limited data)
Verapamil	–	First-line CH profylaxis
TCA	–	No reported AE
Venlafaxine	–	No reported AE
Duloxetine	–	No reported AE
Valproate	Interfere with liver and platelet function	Avoid in women of childbearing age
Topiramate	– Sedation, irritability – Poor suckling, diarrhea	–
Gabapentin	–	No reported AE
Lamotrigine	–	No reported AE
Flunarizine	–	Not recommended: no data available
Lithium	Renal toxicity	Not recommended, but can be considered in uncontrolled CH, refractory to verapamil

(continued)

Table 4.4 (continued)

Medication	Adverse effects	Comments
Botox	–	No reported AE when injected correctly
Nerve blocks	–	No reported AE when injected correctly
Magnesium, riboflavine	–	No reported AE

Adverse effects are the known proven side effects. Concerns cover issues that are presumed based on limited data but for which the causal relationship is not clear

TR1 first trimester, *TR2* second trimester, *TR3* third trimestes, *AE* adverse effects, *ADHD* attention-deficit/hyperactivity disorder, *CM* congenital malformation, *CH* cluster headache, *TCA* tricyclic antidepressants, *ACE-I* ACE inhibitor, *ARB* angiotensin-receptor blocker, *I.V.* intravenously

During breastfeeding period a medication can be considered safe if the relative infant dose is <10% (Table 4.4) [37].

4.3.1 Non-pharmacological Treatment

It is strongly recommended to avoid the well-known triggers like emotional stress, skipping meals, and sleep deprivation. A balanced lifestyle should be encouraged, with particular attention to regular eating, physical activity, and healthy sleeping habits [37, 43, 44].

Acupuncture and behavioral therapies like yoga and biofeedback are safe and can be helpful [37, 44]. Screening for sleep apnea is useful particularly for women with CH, since prevalence is higher in pregnancy and in cluster patients [45].

4.3.2 Symptomatic Treatment

4.3.2.1 Paracetamol/Acetaminophen

Paracetamol is historically considered the safest option and the first choice to treat acute pain during pregnancy and breastfeeding [37, 40, 46, 47]. Nevertheless, there are concerns about a possible relationship between prenatal exposure and an increased risk of attention deficit/hyperactivity disorder (ADHD) and asthma in the child which raise some concern [37, 46, 47]. Patients should be warned about the difference between paracetamol and combination drugs containing paracetamol and other substances, like codeine or caffeine.

4.3.2.2 Aspirin

Acetylsalicylic acid (ASA) in low doses is a safe treatment option, but its use should be limited to low doses (<100 mg/day) and only to the first two trimesters. Higher doses and use in the third trimester have been linked to premature closure of the ductus arteriosus and oligohydramnios [40, 46]. Moreover, ASA interferes with platelet function, increasing the risk of neonatal bleeding [48].

The use of ASA during breastfeeding is not recommended because of a potential toxicity and the risk of Reye's syndrome. A potential adverse effect on platelet function in the infant is suspected but remains unclear [37, 46].

4.3.2.3   Caffeine

The use of caffeine in moderate doses is considered safe as demonstrated by the common consumption of caffeine-containing beverages during pregnancy without any reported adverse effects.

However, moderate-to-high daily doses have been associated to miscarriage, low birth weight, and preterm delivery [46, 47]. Combination drugs containing paracetamol, aspirin, and caffeine should be avoided [40].

There are no concerns about a moderate intake of caffeine during breastfeeding [49].

4.3.2.4   Nonsteroidal Anti-inflammatory Drugs

A conscientious use of these drugs is based on the type of nonsteroidal anti-inflammatory drugs (NSAIDs) and the timing of the pregnancy. Some population-based studies reported an association between congenital malformation and prenatal NSAID exposure in the first trimester, but others do not [37, 46, 47]. NSAIDs should be avoided in the third trimester because of an increased risk of complications like premature closure of the ductus arteriosus, cerebral palsy, neonatal intraventricular hemorrhage, and impaired renal function [40, 47]. The pharmacological properties of these drugs are responsible for the increased risk of miscarriage when used close to conception. Nonselective COX inhibitors like ibuprofen, naproxen, and diclofenac are a relative safe choice in the second trimester, while selective COX2 inhibitors are contraindicated during the whole pregnancy period [46].

Nonselective COX inhibitors are compatible with breastfeeding, preferring ibuprofen because of its low excretion in human milk and short elimination half-life. NSAIDs are contraindicated when breastfeeding newborns with jaundice because they can exacerbate the condition [37, 46, 47, 49].

4.3.2.5   Triptans

Considerable data are available on the use of triptans in pregnancy, especially on sumatriptan. Because of their small molecular weight, triptans can pass through the placenta, but the transfer is slow and passive so that only about 15% of maternal dose reaches the fetus after 4 h [50].

A recent meta-analysis concluded that triptans do not lead to increased rates of major congenital malformations [51]. However, the rates of spontaneous abortions were found elevated when compared to healthy controls (OR 3.54) but not with untreated migraineurs [51].

Some concern exists on a potential increased risk of developing externalizing behaviors and behavioral problems like attention deficit and aggression disorders after in utero exposure to triptans, in particular in the first trimester [52].

Exposure to triptans close to conception is associated with a higher risk of atonic uterus and postpartum hemorrhage [51].

Triptans are compatible with breastfeeding since the infant exposure is very low corresponding to 0.5% of maternal dose [37, 47, 49]. However, mothers could be advised to avoid breastfeeding for 24 h after triptans use [49].

4.3.2.6 Oxygen

High flow administered via a non-rebreathing mask is the preferred treatment for pregnant and breastfeeding women with CH. Oxygen is a safe option without adverse effects on the child or the mother [40, 43, 53].

4.3.2.7 Lidocaine

Lidocaine is an option for pregnant women with CH with a poor response to treatment with oxygen [40, 43, 53]. The intranasal formulation is the best choice since it has a better safety profile than the systemic formulations [53].

All formulations of lidocaine are compatible with breastfeeding [43, 49, 53].

4.3.2.8 Corticosteroids

Prednisone and prednisolone are a reasonable alternative for debilitating CH and status migrainosus [43, 46, 53].

The dose should be kept as low as possible, and they should be avoided during first trimester because of some concern about early lung maturation and a slightly increased risk for cleft palate [53].

Oral prednisone and prednisolone are compatible with breastfeeding, but prolonged high-dose therapy should be avoided because it can affect infant growth and development [43, 49]. It is recommended to delay breastfeeding until 2–8 h after intravenous administration [53].

4.3.2.9 Opioids

Weak opioids like tramadol and codeine can be considered when first-line treatments are not sufficient to bring relief [37, 47]. Opioid exposure in first trimester has been associated with a slightly higher risk for spina bifida and cardiac defects [47].

Prolonged use of opioids may lead to medication-overuse headache (MOH) for the mother and dependency with withdrawal syndrome in the newborn [37]. Stronger formulations should be used with particular caution. Narcotics cross the placenta and consequently are contraindicated during third trimester because they can induce fetal bradycardia, respiratory depression, and birth defects [47].

Sporadic use of weak opioids is compatible with breastfeeding, but frequent use of highly dosed opioids may carry the risk of sedation, respiratory depression, and constipation in the infant [37, 47, 49].

4.3.2.10   Ergots and Ergots Alkaloids

Ergots and ergots alkaloids have uterotonic and vasoconstrictive effects and are contraindicated in pregnancy. Moreover, they can induce teratogenic effects including poor cerebral development and intestinal atresia and as well as other serious adverse effects on the fetus like fetal distress and birth defects [37, 40, 47, 48].

Ergots and ergots alkaloids should be avoided during breastfeeding to prevent systemic side effects in the newborn like diarrhea, vomiting, and convulsions. Moreover, these drugs can decrease prolactin secretion reducing the milk production [37, 47, 49].

4.3.2.11   Antiemetics

Antiemetics are relatively safe during pregnancy [15]. Metoclopramide is commonly used during pregnancy without significant fetal side effects and is commonly used during pregnancy without [40, 43, 47]. Chlorpromazine and prochlorperazine taken during the third trimester are associated with an increased risk of neonatal withdrawal or extrapyramidal symptoms [37], domperidone could lead to long QT syndrome [54], and diphenhydramine could induce sedation and apnea after delivery [49].

Doxylamine, histamine H1 receptor antagonists, dicycloverine, phenothiazine pyridoxine, and phenothiazine are not associated with adverse pregnancy outcomes [49].

There are some concerns on the use of ondansetron during pregnancy due to possible teratogenic effect as well as the potential to cause a serotonin syndrome and QT prolongation [37].

Metoclopramide, chlorpromazine, and prochlorperazine should be avoided during breastfeeding [43, 49]. Antiemetics that could induce irritability, sedation, apnea, and extrapyramidal symptoms are possible [37].

4.3.3   Preventative Treatment

4.3.3.1   Antihypertensive Drugs

β-blockers (metoprolol and propranolol) are the first-line treatment for migraine prophylaxis during pregnancy and breastfeeding [37, 46, 47]. They could have some fetal side effects like intrauterine growth retardation, preterm birth, and respiratory distress [37, 46].

The use of β-blockers in the third trimester can induce neonatal effects like bradycardia, hypotension, and hypoglycemia, and newborns need be closely monitored [37, 47]. β-blockers should be tapered off before labor.

β-blockers are safe during breastfeeding because they are excreted in breast milk in very low doses. However, it is important to pay attention in infants with asthma [49]. Metoprolol is usually preferred over propranolol. Drowsiness, weakness, bradycardia, hypotension, and hypoglycemia are possible side effects [37].

Antihypertensive drugs acting on the renin-angiotensin system, like the ACE inhibitor lisinopril or the angiotensin-receptor blocker candesartan, are contraindicated in pregnancy because of a significant fetal risk [37, 47]. Lisinopril is probably compatible with breastfeeding, but there is no specific data available [49]. Candesartan seems probably compatible as well, with special attention for kidney development [49].

In a pregnant or breastfeeding CH patient, verapamil in the lowest effective dose is the first-line preventative treatment [[43, 49, 53] with breastfeeding].

4.3.3.2 Antidepressants

The tricyclic antidepressants (TCA) are the safest second-line option in case of β-blocker contraindication or inefficacy. Amitriptyline is preferred over nortriptyline. There are data suggesting possible teratogenic effects (e.g., cardiovascular or limb abnormalities), but a clear causal relationship is not sure [37, 47, 48]. All antidepressants can induce withdrawal symptoms when used late in pregnancy, but drowsiness and anticholinergic symptoms like constipation or dry mouth may occur [37, 54]. TCA are relatively safe during breastfeeding since the exposure for infants is about 1–2% of maternal dose, and no accumulation is supposed [46, 47, 49].

The serotonin-norepinephrine reuptake inhibitor (SNRI) venlafaxine should be avoided during pregnancy. There is no clear indication of a possible teratogenic or abortifacient effect of duloxetine. No adverse pediatric effects have been reported in the little data on nursing infants of mothers using the SNRIs duloxetine and venlafaxine [40, 46, 49].

4.3.3.3 Antiepileptic Drugs

Valproate is contraindicated during pregnancy and should be avoided in women of childbearing age because of its teratogenic and fetal side effects like neural tube defects and other serious malformations such as cleft palate, cardiac, or urinary tract defects [37, 47, 55]. Valproate transfers to breast milk in very low doses and seems safe when breastfeeding, but monitoring for platelet and liver function in the child is advised [37, 47, 49].

Topiramate should be avoided in pregnancy because its use is associated with an increased risk of low birth weight and cleft lip/palate, especially when taken during the first trimester [37, 46, 56]. Topiramate reaches infant plasmatic level up to 25%

of maternal levels, and newborns need to be monitored for irritability, sedation, poor suckling, diarrhea, and weight loss [47, 49, 56].

Gabapentin is not recommended during pregnancy due to a link with osteological deformities which is suspected [46]. On the contrary, its use seems compatible with breastfeeding [49].

Lamotrigine has a good safety profile compared with other antiepileptic drugs, and it is considered the preferred option for women of childbearing age [57].

Its use during breastfeeding is safe, and no serious adverse effects or cognitive and development alterations have been reported [58].

4.3.3.4 Flunarizine

There are not enough safety data to support the use of calcium channel blockers in pregnancy and breastfeeding [37, 47].

4.3.3.5 Lithium

Lithium in CH should be avoided in pregnancy due to known teratogenic effects that include congenital cardiac malformations and arrhythmias, polyhydramnios, anomalies of the central nervous system and endocrine system, and stillbirth. The use of lithium should be limited to severe CH patients not responding to verapamil but only if the benefit clearly exceeds the possible risk to the fetus [43, 53].

Lithium prescription during breastfeeding is controversial but can be considered in cases of severe uncontrolled CH [43].

4.3.3.6 Botulinum Toxin Type A

There are only few data available and mainly related for its use as cosmetic treatment, but due to its local mechanisms of action, botulinum toxin type A is probably safe during pregnancy [47].

There are no reports for botulinum toxin type A during breastfeeding. However, a transfer to breast milk is not probable due to its high molecular weight [47].

Until well-controlled data will be available, botulinum toxin type A should only be reserved for severe refractory chronic migraine patients [37, 47, 59].

4.3.3.7 Nerve Blocks

Peripheral nerve blocks are considered safe in pregnancy and breastfeeding. Lidocaine is the most frequently used agent. Other agents commonly used are bupivacaine or betamethasone. Some reports suggest that bupivacaine may be associated with fetal cardiotoxicity [37, 43, 60].

4.3.3.8 Dietary Supplements

Magnesium (up to 350 mg/day) is safe during pregnancy, but there are reports of transient neurological symptoms and hypotonia in newborns [54]. Long-term intravenous administration of magnesium can induce bone abnormalities [37]. These findings make chronic use of magnesium during pregnancy controversial [37].

Coenzyme Q10 seems a safe preventative treatment since there are no reports of severe adverse events [37, 44].

Butterbur (*Petasites hybridus*), feverfew (*Tanacetum parthenium*), and high-dose riboflavine are not recommended during pregnancy [37, 47].

Both magnesium and riboflavine are compatible with lactation. About the safety of coenzyme Q10, butterbur, and feverfew, no conclusive data are available [47, 49].

4.3.3.9 Melatonin

Melatonin seems safe during pregnancy. However there are concerns about the effect that administration of exogenous melatonin could have on the development of the postnatal circadian rhythm [43].

Melatonin is physiologically present in breast milk, where it is excreted in a circadian cycle. Melatonin in low doses seems compatible with breastfeeding [49]. Even if supporting data are not available, it can be assumed that the use of exogenous melatonin can negatively influence postnatal sleep patterns and other hormonal cycles [43].

4.4   Headache-Related Complications During Pregnancy

Headache during pregnancy requires particular attention because it can be a symptom of secondary conditions [40]. At the same time, a pre-existing primary headache can influence the course of pregnancy and delivery and increase the risk of complications [48].

4.4.1   Pregnancy Complications in Patients with Migraine

Migraine does not represent a risk factor for negative pregnancy outcome or fetal malformations [2]. However, migraine can be considered an important risk factor for hypertensive and vascular diseases during pregnancy [61].

The main body of evidence about the relationship between migraine and pregnancy complications comes from a retrospective study on 18,345,538 pregnancies in the United States [62]. Migraine was reported by 33,956 (0.2%) of the examined pregnant women. This study found a strong correlation between migraine and vascular diseases, particularly stroke (OR 15.1), myocardial infarction and other heart diseases (OR 2.1), thromboembolic conditions (OR 3.2), hypertension (OR 8.6), and gestational hypertension/preeclampsia (OR 2.3).

Another retrospective study analyzed data from the Hungarian Case-Control System of Congenital Abnormalities [63]. Among a population of 38,151 infants, 713 (1.9%) of them were born from mothers with a migraine diagnosis. Migraine was associated with a 1.4-fold higher risk of preeclampsia, but the risk of congenital malformations was not increased.

An elevated risk for preeclampsia (OR 1.3) was also detected in a retrospective study on 4911 Taiwanese women with migraine [64]. Moreover, this found an elevated risk for preterm birth (OR 1.24) and low birth weight (OR 1.2).

Similar results regarding increased risk for preeclampsia were found in a retrospective study on 180 Iranian pregnant women; a diagnosis of migraine was associated with a 2.7-fold higher risk for developing preeclampsia [65].

An Italian prospective study analyzed the data of 702 pregnant women who were normotensive before gestation; 38.5% of them reporting migraine headache had a 2.8-fold higher risk of developing hypertensive disorders during pregnancy and a 1.9-fold higher risk for giving birth to low birth weight infants [66].

The risk of developing hypertensive disorders is particularly high if other comorbidities are present. For example, the risk of developing gestational hypertension is 2.5-fold higher in patients with migraine and additionally asthma [67]. Also comorbid mood disorders can increase the risk of hypertensive disorders and preterm birth in pregnant women with migraine [68].

The higher incidence of vascular complications associated with migraine could depend on several pathophysiological mechanisms, including endothelial dysfunction, altered vasoreactivity, platelet hyperaggregation, and decreased prostacyclin production [2, 15, 62].

Furthermore, migraine is associated with a higher risk of other pregnancy complications like nausea and hyperemesis gravidarum [63, 69]. Pregnant migraineurs complain significantly more often about anxiety, stress, vital exhaustion, short sleep duration, and excessive daytime sleepiness [68, 70, 71]. Migraine and depression are distinct conditions, but both could present dysfunction in the serotonergic and dopaminergic system [68].

4.4.2   Pregnancy Complications in Patients with Other Primary Headaches

A retrospective study evaluated data from 430 women after delivery, and 126 (29.3%) of them suffered from a primary headache disorder (81 had MO, 12 MA, and 22 TTH) [6]. No differences in malformation rates and APGAR scores (a method that summarize the health of newborns) were found between women with and without primary headaches, regardless of the headache subtype.

However, history of headache seems to significantly correlate with placental abruption (OR 1.6 for MA, 2.1 for MO, and 1.61 for TTH) [72].

Moreover, a prospective study that compared pregnant women with headache to pregnant women without headache found that preterm deliveries occurred significantly more often within the headache group, with no differences between headaches [73].

4.5   Diagnostics of Headache in Pregnancy

In front of a headache occurring in pregnancy, an early differential diagnosis between a primary and secondary form is crucial for the safety of mother and fetus. In fact, if headache is not the disease, that means it is a symptom of another condition that could be potentially life-threatening. During pregnancy, the most common headaches are migraine and TTH. However, there can be disorders first appearing during pregnancy that manifest with symptoms that resemble primary headaches.

The first step for a correct differential diagnosis of headaches is to collect a proper anamnesis. Important information to obtain is the family history of headache, the age of its onset, whether it is a new or pre-existing symptom, a detailed description of episodes, and accompanying symptoms. Knowing that headache was present before pregnancy can help to predict its evolution during or after gestation.

It is also important to investigate the medication intake and possible comorbidities that could trigger or worsen the course of headache.

If there is a suspicion of the symptomatic character of the headache, it is necessary to carry out a neuroimaging, lumbar puncture, and other methods.

There is a lack of data regarding safety to the fetus in contrast agents such as gadolinium, but given the ability to cross the placenta and remain in the amniotic fluid, its use is not recommended [22]. Iodinated contrast may suppress fetal thyroid function, and its use should be avoided as well [37].

A recently published consensus statement by the European Headache Federation (EHF) can drive the choice of the best technical investigation for headache disorders [27].

4.6   Conclusions

The frequent presentation of headache during pregnancy is not surprising considering that it occurs commonly in the general population, especially in females.

The majority of headaches occurring in pregnancy are primary, such as migraine and tension-type headache. Usually women report a marked improvement or even a cessation of their headache during the second and third trimesters of pregnancy, probably depending on reduction in reproductive hormonal fluctuations. Unfortunately, around 10% of pregnant women experience a worsening of symptoms. However, after delivery most headaches quickly return to their pre-pregnancy pattern.

Migraine is a risk factor for pregnancy complications as gestational hypertension and preeclampsia, stroke, thromboembolic events, and cardiac diseases.

Pregnancy determines modifications of maternal physiology that increase the risk of several serious secondary headache disorders that may require urgent investigation and treatment.

This is the case of preeclampsia, eclampsia, CVT, ischemic and hemorrhagic stroke, SAH, RCVS, PRES, pituitary apoplexy, and thunderclap headache, all conditions showing an overlapping clinical presentation. The differential diagnosis in primary and secondary headache requires one or more between brain MRI and MR angiography with contrast, brain CT, ophthalmoscopy, electroencephalography, ultrasound of the vessels of the head and neck, and lumbar puncture.

Pregnancy and lactation restrict the therapeutic options due to the risk that some drugs are dangerous for the fetus and pass in the maternal milk.

Paracetamol is safe in pregnancy, and ibuprofen can be used for a short time in the first and second trimesters. There are increasing data on triptans' safety in pregnancy and lactation, so sumatriptan can be used to treat migraine attacks if other treatments have failed.

The majority of preventative treatments are not recommended or contraindicated during pregnancy. When behavioral treatment for stress management and lifestyle changes are not enough, metoprolol and propranolol can be used as first choice or amitriptyline as second choice for migraine prevention. Botulinum toxin type A is probable safe, but there are not enough data to support its use during pregnancy.

References

1. GBD 2015 Disease and Injury Incidence and Prevalence Collaborators. Global, regional, and national incidence, prevalence, and years lived with disability for 310 diseases and injuries, 1990-2015: a systematic analysis for the Global Burden of Disease Study. Lancet. 2016;388(10053):1545–602.
2. Menon R, Bushnell CD. Headache and pregnancy. Neurologist. 2008;14(2):108–19.
3. Dixit A, Bhardwaj M, Sharma B. Headache in pregnancy: a nuisance or a new sense? Obstet Gynecol Int. 2012;2012:697697.
4. Granella F, Sances G, Zanferrari C, Costa A, Martignoni E, Manzoni GC. Migraine without aura and reproductive life events: a clinical epidemiological study in 1300 women. Headache. 1993;33(7):385–9.
5. Scharff L, Marcus DA, Turk DC. Headache during pregnancy and in the postpartum: a prospective study. Headache. 1997;37(4):203–10.
6. Maggioni F, Alessi C, Maggino T, Zanchin G. Headache during pregnancy. Cephalalgia. 1997;17(7):765–9.
7. Marcus DA, Scharff L, Turk D. Longitudinal prospective study of headache during pregnancy and postpartum. Headache. 1999;39(9):625–32.
8. Granella F, Sances G, Pucci E, Nappi RE, Ghiotto N, Nappi G. Migraine with aura and reproductive life events: a case control study. Cephalalgia. 2000;20(8):701–7.

9. Sances G, Granella F, Nappi RE, Fignon A, Ghiotto N, Polatti F, Nappi G. Course of migraine during pregnancy and postpartum: a prospective study. Cephalalgia. 2003;23(3):197–205.
10. Mattsson P. Hormonal factors in migraine: a population-based study of women aged 40 to 74 years. Headache. 2003;43(1):27–35.
11. Kelman L. Women's issues of migraine in tertiary care. Headache. 2004;44(1):2–7.
12. Ertresvåg JM, Zwart JA, Helde G, Johnsen HJ, Bovim G. Headache and transient focal neurological symptoms during pregnancy, a prospective cohort. Acta Neurol Scand. 2005;111(4):233–7.
13. Melhado EM, Maciel JA Jr, Guerreiro CA. Headache during gestation: evaluation of 1101 women. Can J Neurol Sci. 2007;34(2):187–92.
14. Aegidius K, Zwart JA, Hagen K, Stovner L. The effect of pregnancy and parity on headache prevalence: the Head-HUNT study. Headache. 2009;49(6):851–9.
15. Contag SA, Mertz HL, Bushnell CD. Migraine during pregnancy: is it more than a headache? Nat Rev Neurol. 2009;5(8):449–56.
16. Amir BY, Yaacov B, Guy B, Gad P, Itzhak W, Gal I. Headaches in women undergoing in vitro fertilization and embryo-transfer treatment. Headache. 2005;45(3):215–9.
17. Kvisvik EV, Stovner LJ, Helde G, Bovim G, Linde M. Headache and migraine during pregnancy and puerperium: the MIGRA-study. J Headache Pain. 2011;12(4):443–51.
18. Bending JJ. Recurrent bilateral reversible migrainous hemiparesis during pregnancy. Can Med Assoc J. 1982;127(6):508–9.
19. Wright GD, Patel MK. Focal migraine and pregnancy. Br Med J (Clin Res Ed). 1986;293(6561):1557–8.
20. Goadsby PJ, Goldberg J, Silberstein SD. Migraine in pregnancy. BMJ. 2008;336(7659):1502–4.
21. Turner DP, Smitherman TA, Eisenach JC, Penzien DB, Houle TT. Predictors of headache before, during, and after pregnancy: a cohort study. Headache. 2012;52(3):348–62.
22. Pearce CF, Hansen WF. Headache and neurological disease in pregnancy. Clin Obstet Gynecol. 2012;55(3):810–28.
23. van Vliet JA, Favier I, Helmerhorst FM, Haan J, Ferrari MD. Cluster headache in women: relation with menstruation, use of oral contraceptives, pregnancy, and menopause. J Neurol Neurosurg Psychiatry. 2006;77(5):690–2.
24. Robbins MS, Farmakidis C, Dayal AK, Lipton RB. Acute headache diagnosis in pregnant women: a hospital-based study. Neurology. 2015;85(12):1024–30.
25. Ramchandren S, Cross BJ, Liebeskind DS. Emergent headaches during pregnancy: correlation between neurologic examination and neuroimaging. AJNR Am J Neuroradiol. 2007;28(6):1085–7.
26. Wabnitz A, Bushnell C. Migraine, cardiovascular disease, and stroke during pregnancy: systematic review of the literature. Cephalalgia. 2015;35(2):132–9.
27. Mitsikostas DD, Ashina M, Craven A, Diener HC, Goadsby PJ, Ferrari MD, Lampl C, Paemeleire K, Pascual J, Siva A, Olesen J, Osipova V, Martelletti P, EHF Committee. European Headache Federation consensus on technical investigation for primary headache disorders. J Headache Pain. 2015;17:5.
28. Negro A, Delaruelle Z, Ivanova TA, Khan S, Ornello R, Raffaelli B, Terrin A, Reuter U, Mitsikostas DD, European Headache Federation School of Advanced Studies (EHF-SAS). Headache and pregnancy: a systematic review. J Headache Pain. 2017;18(1):106.
29. Torelli P, Allais G, Manzoni GC. Clinical review of headache in pregnancy. Neurol Sci. 2010;31(Suppl 1):S55–8.
30. Headache Classification Committee of the International Headache Society (IHS). The International Classification of Headache Disorders, 3rd edition (β version). Cephalalgia. 2013;33(9):629–808.
31. Bousser MG, Ferro JM. Cerebral venous thrombosis: an update. Lancet Neurol. 2007;6(2):162–70.
32. Verdelho A, Ferro JM, Melo T, Canhão P, Falcão F. Headache in acute stroke. A prospective study in the first 8 days. Cephalalgia. 2008;28(4):346–54.

33. Schwedt TJ, Dodick DW. Thunderclap stroke: embolic cerebellar infarcts presenting as thunderclap headache. Headache. 2006;46(3):520–2.
34. Linn FH, Rinkel GJ, Algra A, van Gijn J. Headache characteristics in subarachnoid haemorrhage and benign thunderclap headache. J Neurol Neurosurg Psychiatry. 1998;65(5):791–3.
35. Shanmugalingam R, Reza Pour N, Chuah SC, Vo TM, Beran R, Hennessy A, Makris A. Vertebral artery dissection in hypertensive disorders of pregnancy: a case series and literature review. BMC Pregnancy Childbirth. 2016;16(1):164.
36. Calabrese LH, Dodick DW, Schwedt TJ, Singhal AB. Narrative review: reversible cerebral vasoconstriction syndromes. Ann Intern Med. 2007;146(1):34–44.
37. Wells RE, Turner DP, Lee M, Bishop L, Strauss L. Managing migraine during pregnancy and lactation. Curr Neurol Neurosci Rep. 2016;16(4):40.
38. Brewer J, Owens MY, Wallace K, Reeves AA, Morris R, Khan M, LaMarca B, Martin JN Jr. Posterior reversible encephalopathy syndrome in 46 of 47 patients with eclampsia. Am J Obstet Gynecol. 2013;208(6):468.e1–6.
39. Lee VH, Wijdicks EF, Manno EM, Rabinstein AA. Clinical spectrum of reversible posterior leukoencephalopathy syndrome. Arch Neurol. 2008;65(2):205–10.
40. Schoen JC, Campbell RL, Sadosty AT. Headache in pregnancy: an approach to emergency department evaluation and management. West J Emerg Med. 2015;16(2):291–301.
41. Grand'Maison S, Weber F, Bédard MJ, Mahone M, Godbout A. Pituitary apoplexy in pregnancy: a case series and literature review. Obstet Med. 2015;8(4):177–83.
42. Dodick DW, Wijdicks EF. Pituitary apoplexy presenting as a thunderclap headache. Neurology. 1998;50(5):1510–1.
43. Calhoun AH, Peterlin BL. Treatment of cluster headache in pregnancy and lactation. Curr Pain Headache Rep. 2010;14(2):164–73.
44. Airola G, Allais G, Castagnoli Gabellari I, Rolando S, Mana O, Benedetto C. Non-pharmacological management of migraine during pregnancy. Neurol Sci. 2010;31(Suppl 1):S63–5.
45. Mitsikostas DD, Vikelis M, Viskos A. Refractory chronic headache associated with obstructive sleep apnoea syndrome. Cephalalgia. 2008;28(2):139–43.
46. Coluzzi F, Valensise H, Sacco M, Allegri M. Chronic pain management in pregnancy and lactation. Minerva Anestesiol. 2014;80(2):211–24.
47. Amundsen S, Nordeng H, Nezvalová-Henriksen K, Stovner LJ, Spigset O. Pharmacological treatment of migraine during pregnancy and breastfeeding. Nat Rev Neurol. 2015;11(4):209–19.
48. MacGregor EA. Migraine in pregnancy and lactation. Neurol Sci. 2014;35(Suppl 1):61–4.
49. Hutchinson S, Marmura MJ, Calhoun A, Lucas S, Silberstein S, Peterlin BL. Use of common migraine treatments in breast-feeding women: a summary of recommendations. Headache. 2013;53(4):614–27.
50. Hilaire ML, Cross LB, Eichner SF. Treatment of migraine headaches with sumatriptan in pregnancy. Ann Pharmacother. 2004;38(10):1726–30.
51. Marchenko A, Etwel F, Olutunfese O, Nickel C, Koren G, Nulman I. Pregnancy outcome following prenatal exposure to triptan medications: a meta-analysis. Headache. 2015;55:490–501.
52. Wood ME, Lapane K, Frazier JA, Ystrom E, Mick EO, Nordeng H. Prenatal triptan exposure and internalising and externalising behaviour problems in 3-year-old children: results from the Norwegian mother and child cohort study. Paediatr Perinat Epidemiol. 2016;30(2):190–200.
53. Vanderpluym J. Cluster headache: special considerations for treatment of female patients of reproductive age and pediatric patients. Curr Neurol Neurosci Rep. 2016;16(1):5.
54. Cassina M, Di Gianantonio E, Toldo I, Battistella PA, Clementi M. Migraine therapy during pregnancy and lactation. Expert Opin Drug Saf. 2010;9(6):937–48.
55. [No authors listed]. Warning against use of valproate for migraine prevention during pregnancy. Med Lett Drugs Ther. 2013;55(1418):45.
56. Marmura MJ. Safety of topiramate for treating migraines. Expert Opin Drug Saf. 2017;13(9):12141–7.

57. Pariente G, Leibson T, Shulman T, Adams-Webber T, Barzilay E, Nulman I. Pregnancy outcomes following in utero exposure to lamotrigine: a systematic review and meta-analysis. CNS Drugs. 2017;31(6):439–50.
58. Veroniki AA, Rios P, Cogo E, Straus SE, Finkelstein Y, Kealey R, Reynen E, Soobiah C, Thavorn K, Hutton B, Hemmelgarn BR, Yazdi F, D'Souza J, MacDonald H, Tricco AC. Comparative safety of antiepileptic drugs for neurological development in children exposed during pregnancy and breast feeding: a systematic review and network meta-analysis. BMJ Open. 2017;7(7):e017248.
59. Morgan JC, Iyer SS, Moser ET, Singer C, Sethi KD. Botulinum toxin A during pregnancy: a survey of treating physicians. J Neurol Neurosurg Psychiatry. 2006;77(1):117–9.
60. Govindappagari S, Grossman TB, Dayal AK, Grosberg BM, Vollbracht S, Robbins MS. Peripheral nerve blocks in the treatment of migraine in pregnancy. Obstet Gynecol. 2014;124(6):1169–74.
61. Allais G, Gabellari IC, Borgogno P, De Lorenzo C, Benedetto C. The risks of women with migraine during pregnancy. Neurol Sci. 2010;31(Suppl 1):59–61.
62. Bushnell CD, Jamison M, James AH. Migraines during pregnancy linked to stroke and vascular diseases: US population based case-control study. BMJ. 2009;338:b664.
63. Bánhidy F, Acs N, Horváth-Puhó E, Czeizel AE. Pregnancy complications and delivery outcomes in pregnant women with severe migraine. Eur J Obstet Gynecol Reprod Biol. 2007;134(2):157–63.
64. Chen HM, Chen SF, Chen YH, Lin HC. Increased risk of adverse pregnancy outcomes for women with migraines: a nationwide population-based study. Cephalalgia. 2010;30(4):433–8.
65. Simbar M, Karimian Z, Afrakhteh M, Akbarzadeh A, Kouchaki E. Increased risk of pre-eclampsia (PE) among women with the history of migraine. Clin Exp Hypertens. 2010;32(3):159–65.
66. Facchinetti F, Allais G, Nappi RE, D'Amico R, Marozio L, Bertozzi L, Ornati A, Benedetto C. Migraine is a risk factor for hypertensive disorders in pregnancy: a prospective cohort study. Cephalalgia. 2009;29(3):286–92.
67. Czerwinski S, Gollero J, Qiu C, Sorensen TK, Williams MA. Migraine-asthma comorbidity and risk of hypertensive disorders of pregnancy. J Pregnancy. 2012;2012:22–4.
68. Cripe SM, Sanchez S, Lam N, Sanchez E, Ojeda N, Tacuri S, Segura C, Williams MA. Depressive symptoms and migraine comorbidity among pregnant Peruvian women. J Affect Disord. 2010;122:149–53.
69. Pakalnis A. Migraine and hormones. Semin Pediatr Neurol. 2016;23(1):92–4.
70. Williams MA, Aurora SK, Frederick IO, Qiu C, Gelaye B, Cripe SM. Sleep duration, vital exhaustion and perceived stress among pregnant migraineurs and non-migraineurs. BMC Pregnancy Childbirth. 2010;10:72.
71. Qiu C, Frederick IO, Sorensen T, Aurora SK, Gelaye B, Enquobahrie DA, Williams MA. Sleep disturbances among pregnant women with history of migraine: a cross-sectional study. Cephalalgia. 2015;35(12):1092–102.
72. Sanchez SE, Williams MA, Pacora PN, Ananth CV, Qiu C, Aurora SK, Sorensen TK. Risk of placental abruption in relation to migraines and headaches. BMC Womens Health. 2010;10:30.
73. Marozio L, Facchinetti F, Allais G, Nappi RE, Enrietti M, Neri I, Picardo E, Benedetto C. Headache and adverse pregnancy outcomes: a prospective study. Eur J Obstet Gynecol. 2012;161(2):140–3.

Chapter 5
Migraine and Use of Combined Hormonal Contraception

Francesca Pistoia and Simona Sacco

5.1 Introduction

Migraine onset and activity in women are influenced by the fluctuations of sex hormone levels, particularly estrogen. According to the "estrogen withdrawal hypothesis," migraine episodes are precipitated by a decline in estrogen, as may occur in the menstrual period [1]. Therefore, exogenous estrogens such as those contained in combined hormonal contraceptives (CHC) might interfere with the course of headache in women with migraine. In most cases, the use of CHC leads to an exacerbation or even a new onset of migraine, while in other cases, CHC can lead to an improvement or even be used as migraine prophylaxis (e.g., menstrual migraine [MM]). A complex and still unknown interaction between the vascular actions of estrogens and the vascular alterations of subjects with migraine may also explain the highly increased risk of cardiovascular events among women with migraine using CHC [2].

In the present chapter, we will briefly review the mechanism of action of CHC and the main indications for use, with a focus on health benefits and concerns associated with their prescription, the impact of CHC use on the vascular profile of patients with special attention being paid to the enhanced risk of cardiovascular and cerebrovascular diseases, the interplay between migraine and CHC use, and the use of CHC as therapeutic option for migraine prophylaxis. At the end of the chapter, we will synthesize the findings of the main studies addressing the relationship between CHC use and migraine and will outline recommendations for clinical practice and future research.

F. Pistoia · S. Sacco (✉)
Department of Applied Clinical Sciences and Biotechnology, University of L'Aquila, L'Aquila, Italy
e-mail: francesca.pistoia@univaq.it; simona.sacco@univaq.it

© Springer Nature Switzerland AG 2019
A. Maassen van den Brink, E. A. MacGregor (eds.), *Gender and Migraine*,
Headache, https://doi.org/10.1007/978-3-030-02988-3_5

5.2   Mechanism of Action, Expected Benefits, and Risks

The implementation of CHC as contraceptive agents moved from the observation that, during pregnancy, the ovulation is suppressed through the action of progesterone. This leads to the development of synthetic progestins to be used as *anovulatory* drugs. During the first human trial on the effects of progestins, an accident contamination of the targeted drug with mestranol, a synthetic estrogen, occurred and resulted in a breakthrough bleeding. This paved the way for the later development of combined estrogen-progestin oral contraceptives [3].

The main site of action of CHC is at the hypothalamic and the pituitary level, where CHC exert an inhibitory effect ultimately resulting in a decreased pituitary secretion of both follicle-stimulating hormone (FSH) and luteinizing hormone (LH). This causes the inhibition of follicular development, which prevents ovulation and the formation of the corpus luteum, with the ensuing reduction of ovarian estradiol secretion and the absence of progesterone production. Although ovulation may be inhibited also by the isolated administration of estrogens or progestins, the combined administration of the two compounds increases their antigonadotropic effects [4].

Moreover, it is noteworthy to stress that CHC also offer health benefits beyond contraception. They are considered useful as therapeutic agents in several clinical conditions including dysmenorrhea, menorrhagia, hyperandrogenism, functional ovarian cysts, endometriosis, premenstrual syndrome, myomas, pelvic inflammatory disease, osteoporosis, benign breast disease, and endometrial/ovarian and colorectal cancer [5, 6]. Specifically, symptoms of heavy menstrual bleeding and dysmenorrhea as well as signs of hyperandrogenism such as acne, hirsutism, and polycystic ovary syndrome are significantly reduced by the use of CHC, with a relevant impact on well-being and daily productivity of women [7]. Improved signs of hyperandrogenism are mainly obtained through an increased liver synthesis of the sex hormone-binding globulin (SHBG) ultimately resulting in a decrease of free testosterone levels [5]. Similarly, long-term use of CHC seems to protect against benign breast diseases like breast ductal hyperplasia, fibrocystic breast disease, and fibroadenoma [8]. With respect to cancer, noncontraceptive use of CHC has been reported to provide substantial protection from ovarian and endometrial cancer as well as from colorectal cancer, with a risk reduction being generally greater with longer duration of use [8, 9]. On the other hand, a slightly increased risk for cervical cancer, breast cancer, and liver cancer has been reported in CHC users as compared to nonusers [9].

All together these observations suggest that CHC provide a wide range of noncontraceptive benefits to users. Such benefits have to be properly balanced with the potential increase of cardiovascular and cerebrovascular vulnerability in users, in order to maintain the potential benefits of CHC use without incurring the risk of severe vascular injuries. This may be obtained by thoroughly investigating the vascular profile of individual patients, with special attention being paid to the presence of additional vascular risk factors.

5.3 Migraine, CHCs, and Vascular Risk

According to the available studies, migraine, and mostly migraine with aura (MwA), is associated with an increased risk of ischemic stroke [10, 11] and other vascular events [12, 13]. Moreover, the risk of ischemic stroke in migraineurs is further increased by the use of CHCs [14–19]. In this respect, a pioneering case-control study, investigating the risk of stroke in women aged 15–44 years, found that oral CHC use increased the risk of both ischemic and hemorrhagic stroke and that hypertension, active smoking, and migraine also contributed to increase the cumulative risk [14]. However, it is noteworthy to stress that, at the time of the above study, the available CHC formulations contained estrogen in higher doses as compared to the ones used nowadays. In later observational studies, the combination of active smoking, CHC use, and migraine has been reported to carry the highest risk of ischemic stroke in young women [15–19]. These observations were endorsed by a more recent meta-analysis which confirmed that CHC use causes up to a sevenfold increased risk of ischemic stroke among women with migraine [10]. However, quantifying the individual contribution of CHC use to the cumulative risk of ischemic stroke in women with migraine is challenging, as the available studies have heterogeneous designs and only a few investigated to what extent CHCs independently contribute to enhance the overall risk [14, 15, 18–20]. Besides, no studies assessed the contribution of CHC to the increased risk of vascular events, beyond ischemic or hemorrhagic strokes, in migraineurs. This issue, as well as the joint effect of CHCs and migraine in boosting the vascular risk, should be better elucidated. A recent study suggested that the migraine type is a critical element in evaluating the safety of CHC among women with migraine, as a synergistic effect between migraine and CHC use has been reported only for migraine with aura [21].

All together, these observations suggest an increased risk of ischemic stroke among female migraineurs using CHCs and mostly among women with MwA. As a result, a contraindication to the use of CHC in women with migraine with aura is reasonable to be expected [22]. The quantitative results of the main studies assessing the independent contribution of CHC to the risk of ischemic stroke in women with migraine are summarized in Table 5.1.

5.4 The Effect of CHCs on the Course of Migraine

Early observations, dating back to the 1960s and 1970s, found a link between CHC use and migraine exacerbation [21, 25, 26] and highlighted the association between the development of a new-onset migraine and CHC in 10% of the CHC users [27]. In this respect, an early trial, investigating the effects of CHC containing 50 μg of ethinylestradiol (EE) and 500 μg of levonorgestrel in 40 CHC users as compared to nonusers, found an increased burden of headache in CHC users [28]. Following these preliminary findings, the prescription of CHCs became more cautious in

Table 5.1 Quantitative estimates of the risk of stroke according to CHC use and migraine status

Stroke subtypes	Factors	Effect estimate[a]
Ischemic stroke	CHC use (among women with any migraine)	2.1 [18]
	CHC use + smoke (among women with migraine with aura)	7.0 [17]
	Any migraine + CHC use	2.7–16.9 ([14, 15, 19, 23])
	Migraine without aura + CHC use	1.8 [20]
	Migraine with aura + CHC use	6.1 [20]
	Any migraine + CHC use + smoke	3.3[24]
	Migraine with aura + CHC use + smoke	10.0 [17]
Hemorrhagic stroke	CHC use (among women with migraine)	2.2 [18]
	Any migraine + CHC use	1.1–2.6 [14, 15]

[a]Relative risk or odds ratio

women with a history of migraine, in the attempt to avoid migraine worsening. However, the proportions of women whose migraine has been reported to worsen, improve, or to not show any changes following the use of CHCs are extremely variable across published observational studies. Indeed, some studies did not find any association between CHC use and migraine occurrence [29, 30]. Interestingly, a cross-sectional large-sample study on this issue found migraine worsening or improving in 32% and 30% of cases, respectively [31].

Several factors account for the heterogeneity of findings addressing the impact of CHC use on migraine onset and course. These factors include the use of nonhomogeneous criteria to diagnose migraine, the lack of nonuniform definitions to refer to migraine worsening or improvement, and the different doses of estrogen used, with a progressive decrease in estrogen dose being observed over time [32]. With respect to diagnostic criteria, the crucial element accounting for the above variability lies with the fact that not all the studies investigating the association between CHC use and migraine behavior used the International Classification of Headache Disorders (ICHD) criteria for the diagnosis of migraine. In some studies, the collection of data was based on self-estimated measures, including diaries and face-to-face interviews, thus incurring the risk of misdiagnoses or underestimation/overestimation of the real clinical status and severity. Moreover, it is noteworthy to remind that, over time, the diagnostic criteria for migraine, according to the ICHD, changed [33–35]. However, it is unlikely that such changes have significantly influenced the perception we have about the association between migraine and CHC use. Finally, some individual factors may play a role in modulating the effects of estrogens on migraine; among those factors, genetic polymorphisms in the estrogen receptor genes are the most widely studied, as it is known that some isoforms of estrogen receptors confer an increased susceptibility to suffer from migraine [36].

Regarding the different doses of estrogen used, it has been hypothesized that these can play a relevant role in determining the exacerbation of migraine associated with CHC use, with the highest doses carrying the highest risk. Therefore, the most recent CHC formulations, containing low doses of estrogen, may have a lower impact on migraine worsening as compared to the older higher dose ones. This dose-related effect has been endorsed by a study reviewing the evidence from nine clinical trials involving 43,607 CHC users containing 30 µg ethinylestradiol (EE): headache was reported in 5% of cases [37], higher than 2% rate found with a 20 µg EE dose [38]. However, the lack of standard diagnostic criteria in the assessment of migraine, which was mainly detected through self-reported measures, prompted caution in the interpretation of such results. This became even more evident when a later large community-based study, adopting definite diagnostic criteria for migraine diagnosis, did not find any dose relationship between the amount of estrogen contained in the CHC formulations and the presence of migraine [39]. Similarly, a more recent systematic review failed to demonstrate a lower occurrence of migraine among low-dose CHC users as compared to higher-dose CHC users [40]. Controversial findings have been summarized in a systematic review showing the high variability of effects exerted by CHC use on migraine, with a better safety profile of low-dose estrogen formulations (20–30 µg EE) [41]. However, the issue is still controversial as endorsed by some recent observations suggesting a lower impact of low-dose estrogen formulations on migraine course and a high rate of migraine improvement among women using a combination of low-dose EE and drospirenone [31].

Studies assessing the different impact of CHC use on the course of different migraine subtypes also reported conflicting results. An early retrospective clinic-based study involving 268 women with migraine found that migraine started with CHC use in 16.2% of women diagnosed with MwoA and in 22.2% of women diagnosed with MwA [42]; concerning the evolution of the disease, MwA and MwoA have been reported to have a similar risk of exacerbation following CHC use [42]. On the other hand, a later retrospective study involving 299 CHC users with migraine found a CHC-related migraine worsening particularly in women with menstrual migraine (MM) or MwoA [43], in contrast to other studies showing a high rate of migraine exacerbation in CHC users with MwA as compared to those with MwoA (56.4% vs. 25.3%) [44]. More recent observational data showed a high rate of CHC-related worsening in 69.1% of women with MwA and in 25.4% of women with MwoA [31]. Those conflicting results can be attributed to the already mentioned heterogeneity in the methodology used across different studies.

How different routes of CHC administration may differently influence the migraine course is another matter of debate. CHCs are available not only in the oral form but also as vaginal rings or transdermal patches. The last may reduce the fluctuations of blood estrogen doses and therefore have a positive impact on migraine course as compared to the oral administration. Notably, none of the available studies directly assessed the impact on migraine of different routes of CHC administration, as they only assessed "headache" as a side effect of CHC administration [45]. Open-label trials found no difference in the prevalence of headache when comparing oral CHCs with transdermal patches [46, 47], while the use of vaginal rings has been reported to have a similar impact on headache as compared to oral CHCs containing ≤30 µg EE [48–50] and a better safety profile, resulting in a lower proportion of headache worsening, when compared to oral CHCs containing >30 μg EE [51]. However, it is worth mentioning that non-oral formulations have been compared with intermittent regimens of oral CHCs, while a comparison between non-oral CHC formulations with continuous regimens of oral CHCs is not available.

The course of MM is different in women using CHCs as compared to nonusers, as MM episodes usually occur before the bleeding event in CHC users and after the start of bleeding in nonusers [52, 53]; this is a possible reason to start short-term prophylaxis just after CHC withdrawal in CHC users with MM, while short-term prophylaxis can be started after bleeding in women with MM who do not use CHCs [53].

5.5   CHCs as Migraine Prophylaxis

CHCs may be used as prophylactic agents to prevent estrogen withdrawal in MM. However, randomized controlled clinical trials did not confirm the effectiveness of such agents in MM, resulting in lack of consensus on their real usefulness [54]. CHC administration has been considered useful to limit the fluctuations of blood estrogen levels and to reduce the frequency of migraine episodes triggered by a decline in estrogen level. Estrogen-based preventive strategies include the use of extended-cycle CHCs and estrogen supplementation during the estrogen withdrawal associated with the menstrual phase [55].

Extended-cycle CHCs are aimed at eliminating the 7-day placebo interval which usually follows the 21-day administration of CHCs. Several studies compared the effects of traditional and extended-cycle CHCs on migraine and highlighted the beneficial effects of extended-cycle agents as compared to the traditional ones [56]. Moreover, a retrospective study found extended-cycle approaches being beneficial in MM, due to their capacity to decrease the risk of migraine chronification and of medication overuse [57]. Later interventional studies revealed how a regimen of 24 days of CHC administration followed by 4 days of placebo [58, 59] or a continuous 168-day regimen of CHCs [60, 61] significantly reduces the burden of MM. The dose of estrogen in the 168-day regimen was as low as 30 μg [61], and, as a result, it could be considered suitable also for MwA as suggested by a retrospective case review assessing the effectiveness of a vaginal ring CHC [62]. Finally, an epidemiological survey showed that CHC-induced amenorrhea significantly reduced the burden of MM among women [63]. Although the available evidence supports the effectiveness of extended-cycle CHCs for the prophylaxis of MM, the different studies employed heterogeneous types of hormones administered during different time lengths [64]. The current extended-cycle, low-estrogen options for the hormonal prophylaxis of MM include monthly, extended, and annual oral doses, together with vaginal rings to be inserted monthly [65]. According to expert opinions, also usual oral CHCs might be used as a prophylaxis for MM advising women not to withdraw CHC administration during what would otherwise be the placebo period [65].

Table 5.2 Combined hormonal contraceptive options and their effect on migraine

Type of CHC	Effect
Oral—≥30 µg EE	Increased prevalence of headache in migraineurs mostly in early reports [21, 26] confirmed in more recent studies [39]
Oral—<30 µg EE	Possible better safety compared with CHCs with higher doses of EE [31, 41]; further evidence needed [39, 40]
Oral—extended cycle	Possible beneficial effect on menstrual migraine [58–61]; optimal dose unknown
Oral—usual formulation plus estrogen add back	Possible prophylaxis for menstrual migraine [66]
Transdermal patch	No study directly assessing the impact on migraine; similar prevalence of headache compared with oral CHCs [46, 47]
Vaginal ring	No study directly assessing the impact on migraine; similar prevalence of headache compared with low-dose EE oral CHCs [48–50]

As an alternative to extended-cycle contraception, some researchers have proposed the so-called estrogen add-back, i.e., the administration of estrogen during the placebo period of CHC cycles. The rationale of that approach is the same of extended-cycle CHCs, that is, limiting the estrogen drop during the menstrual period of the ovarian cycle. An open-label study found a mean 77.9% in the number of monthly headache days in 11 women with menstrual-associated migraine treated with a CHC containing 20 µg EE on days 1–21, supplemented with 0.9 mg conjugated equine estrogens on days 22–28 [66], suggesting a potential role of estrogen add-back therapy in women with MM and using CHCs.

CHC formulations contain estrogens combined with variable formulations of progestins. To date, it is unclear whether the type of progestin matters when addressing the potential preventive role of CHCs in MM [65]; a diary-based pilot study suggested the use of dienogest, combined with estradiol valerate for six cycles as the most advisable CHC option in women with MM [67].

A summary of the available evidence about the impact on migraine of the different CHC formulations is provided in Table 5.2.

5.6 Conclusions and Recommendations

According to observational data, migraine may be regarded as an estrogen-sensitive primary headache [31]; therefore, drugs acting on estrogen levels, including CHCs, may either worsen or ameliorate the clinical course of migraine. However, the potential therapeutic applications of CHCs for migraine, and mostly for MM, are currently limited by evidence about the increased risk of stroke among young CHCs users, ultimately resulting in a contraindication to CHCs use in women with MwA [22].

The impact of CHC use on the course of migraine is still controversial: this is mainly due to the extreme variability of studies addressing this issue with respect to the research design, the targeted population, and the methods and criteria used to diagnose migraine. Moreover, available observational studies often put together different types of migraineurs such as subjects with MM, subjects with non-menstrually related migraine, subjects with MwA or MwoA, and women using a wide range of different CHC formulations. This makes difficult drawing definitive conclusions about the effect of CHC of migraine onset and evolution. In order to improve the health of women with migraine, future epidemiological research should focus on the associations of single CHC formulations and specific migraine subtypes; moreover, physicians prescribing CHCs in their daily clinical practice should strictly follow the course of headache in migraineurs, also taking into account that headache may progressively improve in the months following the CHC starting [41]. Therefore, an exacerbation of migraine in a woman using CHC may prove itself to be temporary and cease after 5–6 months of CHC use.

The estrogen withdrawal hypothesis supposes that the drop in blood estrogen doses may cause migraine episodes. Therefore, according to that hypothesis: (1) CHCs with high estrogen doses may exacerbate migraine because they sharpen the estrogen drop after each cycle of CHC use; (2) CHCs with low estrogen doses may have a positive effect on migraine as they may decrease the estrogen drop at the end of CHC cycle; and (3) extended-cycle CHCs may prevent MM as they regularize blood estrogen levels compared with the normal menstrual cycles. Effective therapeutic options include shortening placebo days or choosing a continuous regimen, typically three consecutive packs of active pills followed by a pill-free interval [61]; however, no evidence-based recommendation can be given, to date, for the hormonal management of MM or migraine in general. Besides, those hormonal therapeutic approaches may lead to irregular bleeding [54].

Precaution principles suggest contraindicating the use of CHCs in women with MwA and in those with MwoA and additional risk factors requesting contraception [22]; however, some flaws of currently available studies should be considered. Firstly, the majority of those studies assessed the effect of high-dose estrogen formulations, while recent ones are mostly based upon low-dose estrogen; secondly, the populations included heterogeneous populations of women with migraine. For those reasons, the exact impact of CHCs on the vascular risk of women with migraine might be reassessed, and the use of CHCs might not necessarily be discarded in women with MwA. Further research is needed to assess which CHC formulations will give harm or benefit to women with specific migraine subtypes.

References

1. Somerville BW. The role of estradiol withdrawal in the etiology of menstrual migraine. Neurology. 1972;22(4):355–65.
2. Sacco S, Ricci S, Degan D, Carolei A. Migraine in women: the role of hormones and their impact on vascular diseases. J Headache Pain. 2012;13(3):177–89.
3. Speroff L, Darney P. The history of contraception. In: Speroff L, Darney P, editors. A clinical guide for contraception. Philadelphia, PA: Lippincott Williams and Wilkins; 2011. p. 19–35.

4. Rivera R, Yacobson I, Grimes D. The mechanism of action of hormonal contraceptives and intrauterine contraceptive devices. Am J Obstet Gynecol. 1999;181(5):1263–9.
5. Brynhildsen J. Combined hormonal contraceptives: prescribing patterns, compliance, and benefits versus risks. Ther Adv Drug Saf. 2014;5(5):201–13.
6. Caserta D, Ralli E, Matteucci E, Bordi G, Mallozzi M, Moscarini M. Combined oral contraceptives: health benefits beyond contraception. Panminerva Med. 2014;56(3):233–44.
7. Wasiak R, Filonenko A, Vanness DJ, Wittrup-Jensen KU, Stull DE, Siak S, Fraser I. Impact of estradiol-valerate/dienogest on work productivity and activities of daily living in European and Australian women with heavy menstrual bleeding. Int J Womens Health. 2012;4:271–8.
8. Schindler AE. Non-contraceptive benefits of oral hormonal contraceptives. Int J Endocrinol Metab. 2013;11(1):41–7.
9. Cogliano V, Grosse Y, Baan R, Straif K, Secretan B, El Ghissassi F. WHO International Agency for Research on Cancer. Carcinogenicity of combined oestrogen-progestagen contraceptives and menopausal treatment. Lancet Oncol. 2005;6(8):552–3.
10. Schürks M, Rist PM, Bigal ME, Buring JE, Lipton RB, Kurth T. Migraine and cardiovascular disease: systematic review and meta-analysis. BMJ. 2009;339:b3914.
11. Spector JT, Kahn SR, Jones MR, Jayakumar M, Dalal D, Nazarian S. Migraine headache and ischemic stroke risk: an updated meta-analysis. Am J Med. 2010;123(7):612–24.
12. Sacco S, Ornello R, Ripa P, Pistoia F, Carolei A. Migraine and hemorrhagic stroke: a meta-analysis. Stroke. 2013;44(11):3032–8.
13. Sacco S, Pistoia F, Degan D, Carolei A. Conventional vascular risk factors: their role in the association between migraine and cardiovascular diseases. Cephalalgia. 2015;35(2):146–64.
14. Collaborative Group for the Study of Stroke in Young Women. Oral contraceptives and stroke in young women: associated risk factors. JAMA. 1975;231(7):718–22.
15. Chang CL, Donaghy M, Poulter N. Migraine and stroke in young women: case–control study. The World Health Organization collaborative study of cardiovascular disease and steroid hormone contraception. BMJ. 1999;318(7175):13–8.
16. Haapaniemi H, Hillbom M, Juvela S. Lifestyle-associated risk factors for acute brain infarction among persons of working age. Stroke. 1997;28(1):26–30.
17. MacClellan LR, Giles W, Cole J, Wozniak M, Stern B, Mitchell BD, Kittner SJ. Probable migraine with visual aura and risk of ischemic stroke: the Stroke Prevention in Young Women Study. Stroke. 2007;38(9):2438–45.
18. Schwartz SM, Petitti DB, Siscovick DS, Longstreth WT Jr, Sidney S, Raghunathan TE, Quesenberry CP Jr, Kelaghan J. Stroke and use of low-dose oral contraceptives in young women: a pooled analysis of two US studies. Stroke. 1998;29(11):2277–84.
19. Tzourio C, Tehindrazanarivelo A, Iglésias S, Alpérovitch A, Chedru F, d'Anglejan-Chatillon J, Bousser MG. Case–control study of migraine and risk of ischaemic stroke in young women. BMJ. 1995;310(6983):830–3.
20. Champaloux SW, Tepper NK, Monsour M, Curtis KM, Whiteman MK, Marchbanks PA, Jamieson DJ. Use of combined hormonal contraceptives among women with migraines and risk of ischemic stroke. Am J Obstet Gynecol. 2017;216(5):489.e1–7.
21. Kudrow L. The relationship of headache frequency to hormone use in migraine. Headache. 1975;15(1):36–40.
22. Sacco S, Merki-Feld GS, Ægidius KL, Bitzer J, Canonico M, Kurth T, Lampl C, Lidegaard Ø, Anne MacGregor E, MaassenVanDenBrink A, Mitsikostas DD, Nappi RE, Ntaios G, Sandset PM, Martelletti P. European Headache Federation (EHF) and the European Society of Contraception and Reproductive Health (ESC). Hormonal contraceptives and risk of ischemic stroke in women with migraine: a consensus statement from the European Headache Federation (EHF) and the European Society of Contraception and Reproductive Health (ESC). J Headache Pain. 2017;18(1):108.
23. Milhaud D, Bogousslavsky J, van Melle G, Liot P. Ischemic stroke and active migraine. Neurology. 2001;57(10):1805–11.
24. Lidegaard O. Decline in cerebral thromboembolism among young women after introduction of low-dose oral contraceptives: an incidence study for the period 1980–1993. Contraception. 1995;52(2):85–92.

25. Dalton K. Migraine and oral contraceptives. Headache. 1976;15(4):247–51.
26. Whitty CW, Hockaday JM, Whitty MM. The effect of oral contraceptives on migraine. Lancet. 1966;1(7442):856–9.
27. Larsson-Cohn U, Lundberg PO. Headache and treatment with oral contraceptives. Acta Neurol Scand. 1970;46(3):267–78.
28. Ryan RE. A controlled study of the effect of oral contraceptives on migraine. Headache. 1978;17(6):250–2.
29. Couturier EG, Bomhof MA, Neven AK, van Duijn NP. Menstrual migraine in a representative Dutch population sample: prevalence, disability and treatment. Cephalalgia. 2003;23(4):302–8.
30. Rasmussen BK. Migraine and tension-type headache in a general population: precipitating factors, female hormones, sleep pattern and relation to lifestyle. Pain. 1993;53(1):65–72.
31. Machado RB, Pereira AP, Coelho GP, Neri L, Martins L, Luminoso D. Epidemiological and clinical aspects of migraine in users of combined oral contraceptives. Contraception. 2010;81(3):202–8.
32. Massiou H, MacGregor EA. Evolution and treatment of migraine with oral contraceptives. Cephalalgia. 2000;20(3):170–4.
33. Headache Classification Committee of the International Headache Society. Classification and diagnostic criteria for headache disorders, cranial neuralgias and facial pain. Cephalalgia. 1988;8(Suppl 7):1–96.
34. Headache Classification Subcommittee of the International Headache Society. The International Classification of Headache Disorders: 2nd edition. Cephalalgia. 2004;24(Suppl 1):9–160.
35. Headache Classification Committee of the International Headache Society (IHS). The International Classification of Headache Disorders, 3rd edition. Cephalalgia. 2018;38(1):1–211.
36. Colson NJ, Lea RA, Quinlan S, MacMillan J, Griffiths LR. Investigation of hormone receptor genes in migraine. Neurogenetics. 2005;6(1):17–23.
37. Fotherby K. Twelve years of clinical experience with an oral contraceptive containing 30 micrograms ethinyloestradiol and 150 micrograms desogestrel. Contraception. 1995;51(1):3–12.
38. Fotherby K. Clinical experience and pharmacological effects of an oral contraceptive containing 20 micrograms estrogen. Contraception. 1992;46(5):477–88.
39. Aegidius K, Zwart JA, Hagen K, Schei B, Stovner LJ. Oral contraceptives and increased headache prevalence: the Head-HUNT Study. Neurology. 2006;66(3):349–53.
40. Gallo MF, Nanda K, Grimes DA, Lopez LM, Schulz KF. 20 µg versus >20 µg estrogen combined oral contraceptives for contraception. Cochrane Database Syst Rev. 2013;(8):CD003989.
41. Loder EW, Buse DC, Golub JR. Headache as a side effect of combination estrogen-progestin oral contraceptives: a systematic review. Am J Obstet Gynecol. 2005;193(3):636–49.
42. Cupini LM, Matteis M, Troisi E, Calabresi P, Bernardi G, Silvestrini M. Sex-hormone-related events in migrainous females. A clinical comparative study between migraine with aura and migraine without aura. Cephalalgia. 1995;15(2):140–4.
43. Mueller L. Predictability of exogenous hormone effect on subgroups of migraineurs. Headache. 2000;40(3):189–93.
44. Granella F, Sances G, Pucci E, Nappi RE, Ghiotto N, Nappi G. Migraine with aura and reproductive life events: a case control study. Cephalalgia. 2000;20(8):701–7.
45. MacGregor EA. Contraception and headache. Headache. 2013;53(2):247–76.
46. Audet MC, Moreau M, Koltun WD, Waldbaum AS, Shangold G, Fisher AC, Creasy GW, ORTHO EVRA/EVRA 004 Study Group. Evaluation of contraceptive efficacy and cycle control of a transdermal contraceptive patch vs an oral contraceptive: a randomized controlled trial. JAMA. 2001;285(18):2347–54.
47. Urdl W, Apter D, Alperstein A, Koll P, Schönian S, Bringer J, Fisher AC, Preik M, ORTHO EVRA/EVRA 003 Study Group. Contraceptive efficacy, compliance and beyond: factors related to satisfaction with once-weekly transdermal compared with oral contraception. Eur J Obstet Gynecol Reprod Biol. 2005;121(2):202–10.
48. Ahrendt HJ, Nisand I, Bastianelli C, Gómez MA, Gemzell-Danielsson K, Urdl W, Karskov B, Oeyen L, Bitzer J, Page G, Milsom I. Efficacy, acceptability and tolerability of the combined contraceptive ring, NuvaRing, compared with an oral contraceptive containing 30 microg of ethinyl estradiol and 3 mg of drospirenone. Contraception. 2006;74(6):451–7.

49. Oddsson K, Leifels-Fischer B, de Melo NR, Wiel-Masson D, Benedetto C, Verhoeven CH, Dieben TO. Efficacy and safety of a contraceptive vaginal ring (NuvaRing) compared with a combined oral contraceptive: a 1-year randomized trial. Contraception. 2005;71(3):176–82.
50. Sabatini R, Cagiano R. Comparison profiles of cycle control, side effects and sexual satisfaction of three hormonal contraceptives. Contraception. 2006;74(3):220–3.
51. Stewart FH, Brown BA, Raine TR, Weitz TA, Harper CC. Adolescent and young women's experience with the vaginal ring and oral contraceptive pills. J Pediatr Adolesc Gynecol. 2007;20(6):345–51.
52. Lieba-Samal D, Wöber C, Frantal S, Brannath W, Schmidt K, Schrolnberger C, Wöber-Bingöl C, PAMINA study group. Headache, menstruation and combined oral contraceptives: a diary study in 184 women with migraine. Eur J Pain. 2011;15(8):852–7.
53. Merki-Feld GS, Epple G, Caveng N, Imthurn B, Seifert B, Sandor P, Gantenbein AR. Temporal relations in hormone-withdrawal migraines and impact on prevention- a diary-based pilot study in combined hormonal contraceptive users. J Headache Pain. 2017;18(1):91.
54. Brandes JL. Migraine in women. Continuum (Minneap Minn). 2012;18(4):835–52.
55. Allais G, Chiarle G, Sinigaglia S, Airola G, Schiapparelli P, Bergandi F, Benedetto C. Treating migraine with contraceptives. Neurol Sci. 2017;38(Suppl 1):85–9.
56. Chavanu KJ, O'Donnell DC. Hormonal interventions for menstrual migraines. Pharmacotherapy. 2002;22(11):1442–57.
57. Calhoun A, Ford S. Elimination of menstrual-related migraine beneficially impacts chronification and medication overuse. Headache. 2008;48(8):1186–93.
58. De Leo V, Scolaro V, Musacchio MC, Di Sabatino A, Morgante G, Cianci A. Combined oral contraceptives in women with menstrual migraine without aura. Fertil Steril. 2011;96(4):917–20.
59. Klipping C, Duijkers I, Trummer D, Marr J. Suppression of ovarian activity with a drospirenone-containing oral contraceptive in a 24/4 regimen. Contraception. 2008;78(1):16–25.
60. Coffee AL, Sulak PJ, Hill AJ, Hansen DJ, Kuehl TJ, Clark JW. Extended cycle combined oral contraceptives and prophylactic frovatriptan during the hormone-free interval in women with menstrual-related migraines. J Womens Health (Larchmt). 2014;23(4):310–7.
61. Sulak P, Willis S, Kuehl T, Coffee A, Clark J. Headaches and oral contraceptives: impact of eliminating the standard 7-day placebo interval. Headache. 2007;47(1):27–37.
62. Calhoun A, Ford S, Pruitt A. The impact of extended-cycle vaginal ring contraception on migraine aura: a retrospective case series. Headache. 2012;52(8):1246–53.
63. Vetvik KG, MacGregor EA, Lundqvist C, Russell MB. Contraceptive-induced amenorrhoea leads to reduced migraine frequency in women with menstrual migraine without aura. J Headache Pain. 2014;15:30.
64. Edelman A, Micks E, Gallo MF, Jensen JT, Grimes DA. Continuous or extended cycle vs. cyclic use of combined hormonal contraceptives for contraception. Cochrane Database Syst Rev. 2014;(7):CD004695.
65. Calhoun AH, Batur P. Combined hormonal contraceptives and migraine: an update on the evidence. Cleve Clin J Med. 2017;84(8):631–8.
66. Calhoun AH. A novel specific prophylaxis for menstrual-associated migraine. South Med J. 2004;97(9):819–22.
67. Nappi RE, Terreno E, Sances G, Martini E, Tonani S, Santamaria V, Tassorelli C, Spinillo A. Effect of a contraceptive pill containing estradiol valerate and dienogest (E2V/DNG) in women with menstrually-related migraine (MRM). Contraception. 2013;88(3):369–75.

Chapter 6
Migraine and Use of Progestin-Only Contraception

Gabriele S. Merki-Feld

6.1 Pharmacology of Progestins

Progestins are synthetically synthesized steroid hormones used in contraception and menopausal hormone replacement therapy. They differ in their pharmacologic properties and from progesterone. Progesteroen is released from the ovaries and the corpus luteum after ovulation, and is essential for maintenance of pregnancy and for the transformation of the endometrium. Recent studies indicate that progesterone has a protective effect after traumatic brain injury and stroke and improves neuroregeneration and myelin repair [1–4]. Progesterone and progestins typically act through binding to progesterone receptors, which are widely spread in the brain [5]. In addition, in both sexes the brain contains significant amounts of endogenous progesterone. Most progestins can bind to other steroid receptors as well, such as androgen or estrogen receptors, and exert agonistic or antagonistic actions. The pharmacologic profiles of synthetic progestins also differ. Progesterone influences central neuronal excitability, a key event in migraine pathophysiology [6]. It has been demonstrated that progesterone and some synthetic progestins can antagonize estrogen actions in the reproductive tissues, the brain, and the cultured nerve cells, by lowering estrogen receptor expression [7–9]. Progestin polymorphisms are associated with differences in migraine susceptibility [10]. All these mechanisms could be involved in the effects of desogestrel on migraine, as discussed below.

G. S. Merki-Feld (✉)
Department for Reproductive Endocrinology, University Hospital Zürich, Zürich, Switzerland
e-mail: gabriele.merki@usz.ch

© Springer Nature Switzerland AG 2019
A. Maassen van den Brink, E. A. MacGregor (eds.), *Gender and Migraine*,
Headache, https://doi.org/10.1007/978-3-030-02988-3_6

6.2 Progestin-Only Contraceptives (POCs)

To achieve high contraceptive efficacy, most hormonal contraceptives act by inhibition of ovulation. As unopposed estrogens induce proliferation of the endometrium, combined hormonal contraceptives (CHC) are used with a break to allow scheduled withdrawal bleeding. In predisposed women hormone withdrawal during this break can initiate menstrual migraine.

As detailed before, female migraine is strongly influenced by hormones. Furthermore, migraineurs are exposed to an increased cardiovascular risk [11]. In the context of discussing contraception in migraineurs, not only is the effect of these substances on the course of migraine crucial, but it is also of high importance to prefer methods which do not further increase the individual cardiovascular risk. None of the POC methods are associated with an increase in cardiovascular risk [12].

Most modern progestins inhibit ovulation, so adding an estrogen to a contraceptive is no longer required for contraceptive efficacy. As progestins do not induce proliferation of the endometrium, a pill-free or hormone-free interval to induce withdrawal bleeding is not necessary (Fig. 6.1). In comparison with the natural cycle or CHC use, continuous use of POC results in more continuous and stable hormone levels, which might improve tolerability for migraineurs. Another advantage of POC is that, in contrast to estrogens, progestins do not increase the risk for venous thromboembolism (VTE) or stroke. A disadvantage of POCs is the unpre-

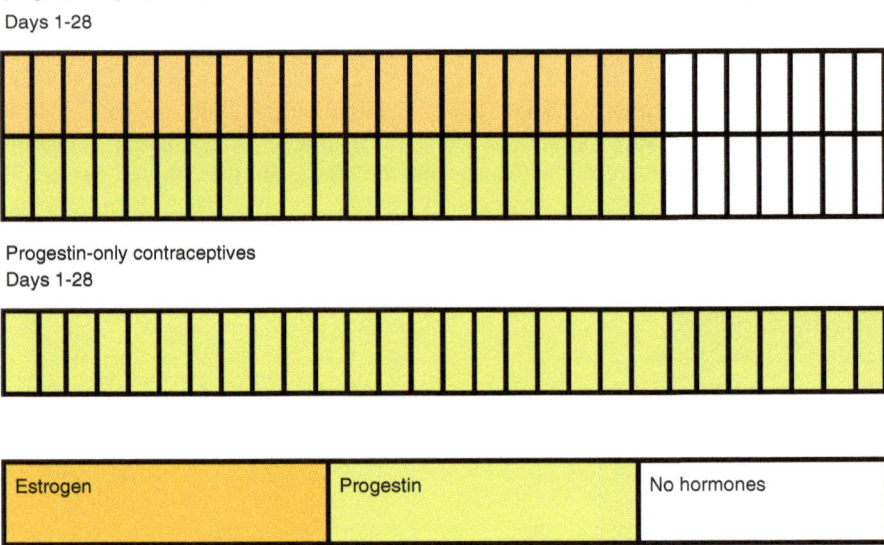

Fig. 6.1 Typical use of combined hormonal contraceptives (CHC) and progestin-only contraceptives

dictable bleeding pattern, ranging from amenorrhea to prolonged spotting. Bleeding is typically light but intolerable for a subset of users. Proactive patient education about changes in bleeding pattern before initiation of POC, as well as supportive follow-up, can markedly reduce these concerns. The frequency and duration of such unscheduled bleeding decrease with increasing duration of use. In contrast to other routes of delivery, intrauterine systems with release of levonorgestrel do not typically inhibit ovulation. Therefore, cyclic hormone fluctuations are only modified and may even be stronger than usual if follicles persist and do not rupture. This implies less stable hormone levels, even if the local levonorgestrel release in the uterus might impede withdrawal bleeding.

6.3 Progestin-Only Methods Available in Most European Countries, Mechanism of Action, and Hormone Fluctuations During Their Use

1. Continuous daily pill with desogestrel 75 μg (POP)
2. Implant releasing etonogestrel
3. Three-monthly injection with depot-medroxyprogesterone acetate (DMPA)
4. Intrauterine systems with release of levonorgestrel (LNG-IUS)

6.3.1 Continuous Daily Pill with Desogestrel 75 μg (POP)

This POP inhibits ovulation and has to be taken continuously. The Pearl index (number of pregnancies in 100 women using this method for a year) for correct use is comparable with that of CHC, 0.3–0.6. As ovulation is inhibited and as there is no hormone withdrawal, this contraceptive seemed to be a good alternative to CHC in women with migraine. The hormone dose is low and allows a basal estradiol production in the ovaries. Therefore, it is of importance to be aware that efficacy can easily be reduced in the situation of co-administration of other substances. Several studies have shown a positive effect of this contraceptive on migraine with and without aura [13–16]. Most frequent adverse events include bleeding problems, weight changes, effects on mood, acne, and headache.

6.3.2 Etonogestrel-Releasing Implant

This single-rod non-biodegradable implant is inserted subdermally under local anesthetic in the medial aspect of a patient's upper arm using a specialized needle applicator. The implant provides highly effective contraception for up to 3 years. Suppression of ovulation is the primary mechanism of this contraceptive method.

As with the POP, the hormone dose of this implant is low and is comparable to the desogestrel POP. Therefore it is of importance to be aware that efficacy can easily be reduced in the situation of co-administration of other substances. Once the etonogestrel contraceptive implant is removed, rapid return of ovulation occurs, and fertility rates are unaffected. The continuous hormone release of the implant contributes to low fluctuations in plasma levels of the substance. Of importance for premenopausal women is that sufficient estrogens are produced in the ovaries. Adverse events include bleeding problems, weight change, acne, effects on mood, and headache.

6.3.3   Depot-Medroxyprogesterone Acetate (DMPA) Injection

DMPA is an injectable, progestin-only contraceptive that provides highly effective, relatively long-acting (3 months), reversible contraception. DMPA is available in two formulations: 150 mg/1 mL for intramuscular (im) injection and 104 mg/0.65 mL for subcutaneous (sc) injection. It can be given every 3 months 12–14 weeks because low solubility of the microcrystals at the injection site allows pharmacologically active drug levels to persist and remain effective for several months. DMPA primarily acts by inhibition of gonadotropin secretion, thereby inhibiting follicular maturation and ovulation. Estrogen production in the ovaries is more suppressed in comparison to the POP or the implant. The endometrium becomes atrophic, and many women develop amenorrhea over longer duration of use. The following side effects were reported by more than 5% of subjects: menstrual irregularities (unscheduled bleeding or amenorrhea), weight changes, headache, and abdominal pain. A number of interactions with other medications are reported. In such a situation, the interval between injections can be shortened.

6.3.4   Intrauterine Systems with Release of Levonorgestrel (LNG-IUS 20)

At present there are three doses of levonorgestrel-releasing IUS available. Only one of these (the LNG-IUS 20 marketed under the name Mirena®) releases enough progestin to reduce significantly the amount of bleeding or induce amenorrhea. Only this device will be discussed in this context, as some clinicians use it to suppress bleeding in women with menstrual migraine. The LNG-IUS 20 provides highly effective contraception for up to 5 years. It suppresses endometrial growth by releasing levonorgestrel into the uterine cavity. Low serum levels of absorbed progestin are mostly below the threshold for inhibition of ovulation, which occurs in 2/3 of the cycles. The LNG-IUS 20 has however an influence on follicular development and growth. Unruptured follicles and ovarian cysts can produce high levels of estrogen, which might impact women susceptible to hormonal headaches. Frequent side effects are ovarian cysts, rare side effects include acne, weight gain, depression, and decreased libido.

6.4 Evidence for Effects of POC on Migraines

Four studies investigated the impact of the POP with desogestrel on migraine [13–15, 17]. No studies have investigated the effect of the implant, DMPA, and LNG-IUS. As a consequence, only clinical observations are discussed here.

6.4.1 Continuous Daily Pill with Desogestrel 75 μg (POP)

A recent meta-analysis concluded that desogestrel 75 μg is associated with a modest reduction in migraine frequency and use of analgesics, but randomized placebo-controlled trials are needed [18]. Four diary-based studies indicate that the use of the progestin-only contraceptive pill with desogestrel results in a reduction in migraine days and migraine intensity within 3 months of use [13]. The use of analgesics is also significantly reduced, and users experience a significant increase in quality of life [14, 19]. Improvement has been observed in patients with migraine with aura and migraine without aura, including non-menstrual migraine [15, 16]. It can only be speculated on possible mechanisms underlying the effects of desogestrel on migraine. One is based on the idea of a direct or receptor-mediated effect of the progestin on the trigeminovascular system. In contrast to estrogens, progesterone seems to attenuate trigeminovascular nociception and to reduce dural plasma protein extravasation following stimulation of the trigeminal ganglion [20–22]. In mice, the thresholds for cortical spreading depression (CSD) are lower in cycling females than in males [22]. This would support the hypothesis that the desogestrel-induced maintenance of low estrogen levels might upregulate the threshold for CSD and thus reduce the number of migraine with aura attacks. Another mechanism underlying the effect of the progestin on headache could be that desogestrel or its metabolite etonogestrel, like progesterone and allopregnanolone, may decrease cortical excitability via the GABA receptor [5, 23, 24].

6.4.2 Implant Releasing Etonogestrel

Etonogestrel is the active metabolite of desogestrel. Therefore, it could be assumed that this contraceptive exerts a similar positive impact on migraine as desogestrel. However, this has never been addressed in scientific studies. In daily clinic, some women express their wish to use a nonoral method because they might feel better protected with a method they do not have to remember daily. In migraineurs who started desogestrel and later changed to the implant, we never observed a worsening of migraine (observation based on limited clinical experience). With regard to the risk for stroke, there is no concern with the implant.

6.4.3   Three-Monthly Injection with Depot Medroxyprogesterone Acetate (DMPA)

No studies investigate the impact of DMPA on migraine. Several reasons support the view that this medication will not have a negative impact on the course of migraine in the majority of users: ovulation is suppressed, estrogen levels are low and stable, and there is no withdrawal, either of estrogen or of progestins. The steroid structure of DMPA differs from that of desogestrel. Therefore, it cannot be assumed that DMPA reduces migraine frequency in general. There might however be a positive effect on withdrawal headaches.

6.4.4   Intrauterine Systems with Release of Levonorgestrel (LNG-IUS 20)

The LNG-IUS 20 can induce amenorrhea by local release of LNG into the uterine cavity. Even if bleeding is suppressed, users experience regular ovulation and estrogen withdrawal at the end of the cycle. A positive effect of this contraceptive on migraine is not to be expected. Studies to investigate this issue have not been performed yet. Some women develop follicular cysts, which cause hormone fluctuations stronger than those occurring in the natural cycle. This might explain the strong increase in migraine days in a subgroup of migraineurs using this device (clinical experience). On the other hand, in some women with pure menstrual migraine, migraine attacks improve by stopping the bleeding (clinical experience).

6.5   Conclusions

POC might be the first choice option for women with migraine who request effective contraception. Desogestrel 75 μg has a positive impact on migraine, in addition to providing contraception in the majority of women. The frequently low tolerability of the LNG_IUS 20 in women with episodic migraine needs to be addressed during counselling.

References

1. Cutler SM, Cekic M, Miller DM, Wali B, VanLandingham JW, Stein DG. Progesterone improves acute recovery after traumatic brain injury in the aged rat. J Neurotrauma. 2007;24(9):1475–86.
2. Wright DW, Kellermann AL, Hertzberg VS, Clark PL, Frankel M, Goldstein FC, et al. ProTECT: a randomized clinical trial of progesterone for acute traumatic brain injury. Ann Emerg Med. 2007;49(4):391–402. e1-2.
3. Hussain R, El-Etr M, Gaci O, Rakotomamonjy J, Macklin WB, Kumar N, et al. Progesterone and Nestorone facilitate axon remyelination: a role for progesterone receptors. Endocrinology. 2011;152(10):3820–31.
4. Xiao G, Wei J, Yan W, Wang W, Lu Z. Improved outcomes from the administration of progesterone for patients with acute severe traumatic brain injury: a randomized controlled trial. Crit Care. 2008;12(2):R61.
5. Schumacher M, Mattern C, Ghoumari A, Oudinet JP, Liere P, Labombarda F, et al. Revisiting the roles of progesterone and allopregnanolone in the nervous system: resurgence of the progesterone receptors. Prog Neurobiol. 2014;113:6.
6. Chauvel V, Schoenen J, Multon S. Influence of ovarian hormones on cortical spreading depression and its suppression by L-kynurenine in rat. PLoS One. 2013;8(12):e82279.
7. Prange-Kiel J, Rune GM, Zwirner M, Wallwiener D, Kiesel L. Regulation of estrogen receptor alpha and progesterone receptor (isoform A and B) expression in cultured human endometrial cells. Exp Clin Endocrinol Diabetes. 2001;109(4):231–7.
8. Aguirre C, Jayaraman A, Pike C, Baudry M. Progesterone inhibits estrogen-mediated neuroprotection against excitotoxicity by down-regulating estrogen receptor-beta. J Neurochem. 2010;115(5):1277–87.
9. Jayaraman A, Pike CJ. Progesterone attenuates oestrogen neuroprotection via downregulation of oestrogen receptor expression in cultured neurones. J Neuroendocrinol. 2009;21(1):77–81.
10. Joshi G, Pradhan S, Mittal B. Role of the oestrogen receptor (ESR1 PvuII and ESR1 325 C->G) and progesterone receptor (PROGINS) polymorphisms in genetic susceptibility to migraine in a North Indian population. Cephalalgia. 2010;30(3):311–20.
11. Buse DC, Reed ML, Fanning KM, Kurth T, Lipton RB. Cardiovascular events, conditions, and procedures among people with episodic migraine in the US population: results from the American Migraine Prevalence and Prevention (AMPP) study. Headache. 2017;57(1):31–44.
12. Roos-Hesselink JW, Cornette J, Sliwa K, Pieper PG, Veldtman GR, Johnson MR. Contraception and cardiovascular disease. Eur Heart J. 2015;36(27):1728–34. 34a-34b.
13. Merki-Feld GS, Imthurn B, Langner R, Sandor PS, Gantenbein AR. Headache frequency and intensity in female migraineurs using desogestrel-only contraception: a retrospective pilot diary study. Cephalalgia. 2013;33(5):340–6.
14. Merki-Feld GS, Imthurn B, Langner R, Seifert B, Gantenbein AR. Positive effects of the progestin desogestrel 75 mug on migraine frequency and use of acute medication are sustained over a treatment period of 180 days. J Headache Pain. 2015;16:522.
15. Morotti M, Remorgida V, Venturini PL, Ferrero S. Progestin-only contraception compared with extended combined oral contraceptive in women with migraine without aura: a retrospective pilot study. Eur J Obstet Gynecol Reprod Biol. 2014;183:178–82.
16. Nappi RE, Sances G, Allais G, Terreno E, Benedetto C, Vaccaro V, et al. Effects of an estrogen-free, desogestrel-containing oral contraceptive in women with migraine with aura: a prospective diary-based pilot study. Contraception. 2011;83(3):223–8.
17. Nappi RE, Merki-Feld GS, Terreno E, Pellegrinelli A, Viana M. Hormonal contraception in women with migraine: is progestogen-only contraception a better choice? J Headache Pain. 2013;14:66.
18. Warhurst S, Rofe CJ, Brew BJ, Bateson D, McGeechan K, Merki-Feld GS, et al. Effectiveness of the progestin-only pill for migraine treatment in women: a systematic review and meta-analysis. Cephalalgia. 2018;38:754.

19. Merki-Feld GS, Imthurn B, Seifert B, Merki LL, Agosti R, Gantenbein AR. Desogestrel-only contraception may reduce headache frequency and improve quality of life in women suffering from migraine. Eur J Contracept Reprod Health Care. 2013;18(5):394–400.
20. Cutrer FM, Moskowitz MA. Wolff Award 1996. The actions of valproate and neurosteroids in a model of trigeminal pain. Headache. 1996;36(10):579–85.
21. Multon S, Pardutz A, Mosen J, Hua MT, Defays C, Honda S, et al. Lack of estrogen increases pain in the trigeminal formalin model: a behavioural and immunocytochemical study of transgenic ArKO mice. Pain. 2005;114(1-2):257–65.
22. Bolay H, Berman NE, Akcali D. Sex-related differences in animal models of migraine headache. Headache. 2011;51(6):891–904.
23. Liu A, Margaill I, Zhang S, Labombarda F, Coqueran B, Delespierre B, et al. Progesterone receptors: a key for neuroprotection in experimental stroke. Endocrinology. 2012;153(8):3747–57.
24. Kokate TG, Svensson BE, Rogawski MA. Anticonvulsant activity of neurosteroids: correlation with gamma-aminobutyric acid-evoked chloride current potentiation. J Pharmacol Exp Ther. 1994;270(3):1223–9.

Chapter 7
Sex Hormones and CGRP

Eloísa Rubio-Beltrán and Alejandro Labastida-Ramírez

7.1 Introduction

Migraine is three times more prevalent in women than in men [1], with female patients presenting also a higher risk of cardiovascular events, including cardiovascular mortality [2]. Moreover, the intensity and frequency of headaches are higher in women, as well as the risk of chronification, which leads to greater disability [1].

The mechanisms behind the sex disparity in migraine are not completely understood, but it is thought to be mediated through changes in ovarian steroid hormones. Somerville was the first to propose this in the 1970s by studying the effect of estradiol withdrawal in the precipitation of migraine attacks and concluded that during the late luteal phase of the menstrual cycle, the decline in estrogen concentrations in plasma correlates with the precipitation of migraine attacks [3]. This was later confirmed by a recent study that showed that women with migraine present a faster decline in (urinary) estrogen levels during the late luteal phase, compared to controls [4]. Furthermore, during the phases of the menstrual cycle that present elevated levels of estrogen, women appear to have a reduction of migraine attacks, suggesting a protective role [5]. Changes in progesterone, however, do not seem to have a protective nor triggering effect on migraine attacks [6].

The previous results are in line with the occurrence of migraine between sexes during the lifetime. Before puberty, migraine prevalence is similar between sexes and after menarche is increased for women in a 3:1 ratio. Interestingly, similar rates are observed in transsexuals undergoing estrogen therapy for male to female transition [7]. Moreover, not only hormonal changes throughout the menstrual cycle have been seen to alter the frequency of migraine attacks but also fluctuations in hormone levels during pregnancy, puerperium, breastfeeding, perimenopause, and menopause

E. Rubio-Beltrán (✉) · A. Labastida-Ramírez
Division of Vascular Medicine and Pharmacology, Department of Internal Medicine, Erasmus Medical Center, Rotterdam, The Netherlands
e-mail: a.rubiobeltran@erasmusmc.nl; a.labastidaramirez@erasmusmc.nl

[4, 8, 9]. Disorders such as menorrhagia, dysmenorrhea, polycystic ovary syndrome, and endometriosis have been related to higher prevalence of migraine [10–12]; and, in contrast, the use of hormone replacement therapy, estrogen receptor antagonists, and contraceptive pills seems to reduce the frequency of migraine by reducing hormonal fluctuations [13, 14].

7.2   Migraine Pathophysiology

Several theories have arisen regarding migraine pathophysiology [15]. Currently, it is considered a neurovascular disorder that involves activation of the trigeminovascular system [16]. This system comprises both peripheral and central projections, the former via the trigeminal ganglion that sends sensory fibers to the dura mater and the cranial vasculature [17] and the latter, via the trigeminocervical complex that consists of the trigeminal nucleus caudalis and the upper two cervical divisions [18]. The activation of this system is considered to be followed by the release of calcitonin gene-related peptide (CGRP) from the sensory fibers, causing vasodilation of the cranial vasculature [19].

7.3   CGRP and Migraine

CGRP is an ubiquitous neuropeptide involved in the modulation of several cardiovascular, neural, immune, and metabolic (patho)physiological processes [20]. It is formed by 37 amino acids, and two isoforms have been described: α-CGRP and β-CGRP [21, 22]. α-CGRP is widely expressed throughout the trigeminovascular system [23, 24], while β-CGRP is mainly expressed in the enteric nervous system [25]; therefore, migraine-related studies focus only on α-CGRP, and in this chapter it will be referred to simply as CGRP, unless stated otherwise. The CGRP receptor complex is formed by three components: the G protein-coupled "calcitonin receptor-like" receptor (CLR), the "receptor activity modifying protein 1" (RAMP1), and the "receptor component protein" (RCP). The presence of these components determines the function of the CGRP receptor complex [20].

As mentioned above, it is considered that during a migraine attack, CGRP is released from the sensory fibers that originate from the trigeminal ganglion, causing neurogenic vasodilation and nociceptive transmission [19, 26]. In accordance with this, studies have shown that during a migraine attack, there is an increase of CGRP levels in plasma in the jugular vein [26], and treatment with triptans normalizes these levels [27]. Also, intravenous infusions of CGRP are known to provoke migraine-like attacks in migraine patients [28]. These studies have led to the development of antibodies against CGRP or its receptor for the treatment of migraine, and so far, all the clinical trials have shown promising results [29–32].

7.4 Sex Hormones and CGRP Studies

In view of the high prevalence of migraine in women and the role of CGRP in migraine pathophysiology, it is important to consider a possible interaction between CGRP signaling and ovarian steroid hormones. Previous studies have already described sex hormone receptors in the trigeminovascular system [33]; however, no studies have achieved to explain the signaling pathways behind this possible interaction. In the following sections, preclinical and clinical studies in migraine models where differences in sex hormones have been observed will be discussed.

7.5 Preclinical Studies

Despite the high prevalence of migraine in women, studies in animals are most often performed in males, in order to reduce the biological variations due to the female cycle [34]. Interestingly, independent from the estrous cycle, female rats present higher mRNA levels of CGRP in the medulla and lower mRNA levels of the CGRP receptor components CLR, RAMP1, and RCP in medulla and trigeminal ganglion [35] when compared to males, suggesting a sex-dependent differential response.

Studies focusing on hormonal fluctuations and CGRP are limited, and the grand majority describes the effects of estrogen. There are three receptors for estrogen: two nuclear (alpha, ERα; beta, ERβ) and one G protein-coupled estrogen receptor (GPER), all of them described throughout the trigeminovascular system (Table 7.1).

Table 7.1 Sex hormone receptors described in the trigeminovascular system in preclinical and clinical studies

Receptor		Dura mater	Cranial blood vessels	Trigeminal ganglion	Trigeminal nerve nuclei
Estrogen	ERα	Rat [36] Human [37]	Rat [38, 39] Human [40]	Mouse [41], rat [42, 43] Human ND	Rat [36, 43, 44] Human [45, 46]
	ERβ	Pig [47] Human [37]	Rat [39] Human [40]	Rat [43] Human ND	Rat [43] Human [45, 46]
	GPER	Rat [36] Human ND	Rat [48] Human ND	Rat [44] Human ND	Rat [36] Human ND
Progesterone receptor		Rat [49] Human [37]	Human [50]	Mouse [51] Human ND	Rat [52] Human ND
Androgen receptor		Rat [53] Human ND	Rat [38] Human [40]	Rat [54] Human ND	Rat [55] Human ND

Taken and modified from [56]

The exact function is not yet completely understood, but it is believed that they modulate CGRP expression, although results are not conclusive. During the estrous cycle, the mRNA levels of CGRP in rat trigeminal nucleus [57] and mouse trigeminal ganglion [41] appear to remain constant. These levels are increased in ovariectomized rats and later normalized with estrogen treatment [42]. Furthermore, reduced levels of estrogens have been seen to increase CGRP expression in the periaqueductal gray area [58]. Likewise, treatment with estrogen decreases CGRP levels in the trigeminal nucleus caudalis [59]. Nevertheless, an increase in estrogen levels not always downregulates CGRP expression, as in the rat pituitary it has been described to be upregulated [60]. Further results in dorsal root ganglion (DRG) [61–64], and the medial preoptic nucleus of the hypothalamus [65, 66], are inconsistent among studies.

An *in vivo* model to study the trigeminovascular mechanisms involved in migraine is the intravital microscopy on a closed cranial window. This model consists on measuring changes in middle meningeal artery diameter induced by exogenous administration of CGRP or by endogenous CGRP (i.e., periarterial electrical stimulation or intravenous capsaicin). In this model, the effect of 17β-estradiol, progesterone, and the combination was studied in ovariectomized rats with and without hormonal replacement [67]. While ovariectomy and hormonal replacement alone did not modify the responses to CGRP, the treatment with 17β-estradiol enhanced the vasodilatory responses induced by electrical stimulation, suggesting a prejunctional modulation of CGRP release by estrogen. In another *in vivo* model, researchers demonstrated that the declining in ovarian steroid hormones observed during the later halves of the proestrus and estrus correlates with an increased sensitization of the trigeminal nucleus caudalis [68], suggesting that the activity of the trigeminovascular system is regulated by the hormonal fluctuations during the estrous cycle.

Studies focused on progesterone and androgen receptors are scarce. Both types of receptors have been described in the dura mater, cranial vasculature, trigeminal ganglion, and trigeminal nerve nuclei [69]. In rats, it has been shown that progesterone decreases CGRP accumulation in the trigeminal nucleus, while testosterone does not modify CGRP levels [57]. In a porcine model, treatment with elevated levels of testosterone downregulated CGRP in the DRG, whereas progesterone treatment increased the levels of CGRP in DRG and plasma [70].

In summary, preclinical studies have shown that ovarian steroid hormones participate in the modulation of the trigeminovascular system activity, as well as in the release and expression of CGRP. Nevertheless, more studies are needed to further elucidate the exact mechanisms behind this modulation, as well as the translation of these results to a clinical perspective.

7.6   Clinical Studies

Migraine attacks have been associated with an increase of CGRP in plasma [26]. Interestingly, when measured in healthy subjects, levels of CGRP are higher in women than in men and even higher in women using contraceptive pills [71]. Also,

CGRP levels are increased during pregnancy, with their peak near term, and they normalize after delivery, while postmenopausal women show a decrease in CGRP concentrations [72, 73]. Some of these results may seem contradictory, since in patients under contraceptives, and during pregnancy and postpartum, a reduction of migraine attacks has been described [9, 13]. This could be explained by the site of venipuncture; in migraine patients, the increased levels of CGRP during attacks have been observed only when measured from jugular blood, while the aforementioned studies measured cubital blood samples. Therefore, it is possible that although CGRP is elevated in the systemic circulation, local CGRP levels in structures relevant to migraine (i.e., cranial vessels) are not increased or that high concentrations of CGRP desensitize the receptor, thus reducing the frequency of attacks.

In clinical research it is important to develop noninvasive techniques. A clear example is the use of laser Doppler perfusion imaging for the study of changes in dermal blood flow (DBF) induced by electrical, chemical, or thermal stimulation of the skin. Previous studies demonstrated that topical application of capsaicin on the forearm activates the transient receptor potential vanilloid type 1 (TRPV1) receptor located in the sensory neurons, resulting in the release of CGRP and vasodilation, reflected as an increase in DBF [74–77]. With this model, the sex differences in CGRP release from the primary sensory neurons were analyzed and further correlated with the levels of estrogen and progesterone [78]. Male healthy volunteers and migraine patients showed stable DBF responses during all the measurements. On the other hand, healthy women presented higher DBF responses during the menstruation phase, and female patients displayed this increase during menstruation and the late secretory phase. No differences in progesterone and estradiol were observed between groups, suggesting an increased sensitivity of the TRPV1 or the CGRP receptors.

As the previous experiments were performed in the forearm, a modification of the model was done in order to assess changes in DBF in vessels innervated by the trigeminal nerve. The ophthalmic nerve (V1), more specifically, the frontal branch, innervates the forehead; therefore, in the new model, topical application of capsaicin or electrical stimulation (i.e., iontophoresis) was performed on the forehead [79]. With this model, the differences in DBF responses mediated by the trigeminal nerve activation were studied in healthy women, patients with menstrually related migraine (MRM), and postmenopausal women [80]. Similar to the results obtained in the forearm model, healthy subjects showed increased responses during the menstruation phase, which had been observed previously in a study where intradermal injections of capsaicin in the forehead induced higher sensory and vasomotor responses, as well as an increase in pain perception during menstruation [81]. Moreover, postmenopausal women presented no changes in DBF responses throughout the measurements. Unexpectedly, MRM patients did not present changes in DBF during their cycle, and their estradiol levels during the luteal phase were lower when compared to healthy subjects. Although the exact mechanisms behind these differences were not explored, it could be explained by a dysfunction in the estrogen-regulated TRPV1 receptor expression in sensory neurons [82].

Another approach for the study of sex differences in the central nervous system of patients with migraine is the use of functional neuroimaging, more specifically, high-field magnetic resonance imaging (MRI). Using this technique, a female migraine patient was followed during a whole month. The subject had an MRI daily, and nociceptive trigeminal stimulation was performed. The researchers found an alteration in the functional coupling with the spinal trigeminal nuclei and the dorsal rostral pons during the preictal day and the pain phase of migraine attacks. Although the study assessed the phases of the menstrual cycle, this was not correlated to the trigeminal activity nor the triggering of migraine attacks [83]. In another MRI study, it was shown that women with migraine present a stronger activation of the spinal trigeminal nucleus, when compared to men [84]; however, as in the previous study, the phase of the menstrual cycle of the participants was not reported. An MRI study where the activation of the trigeminovascular system is correlated with the hormonal fluctuations of the female cycle is required, as it could improve our understanding of migraine pathophysiology and treatment.

Although the sex differences in the trigeminovascular system are clear, it is important to define if hormone fluctuations have a direct action on the vasculature, on the release of CGRP or in the central activation of the trigeminal system. In Fig. 7.1, the structures where estradiol has been described to modulate the trigeminovascular system are represented.

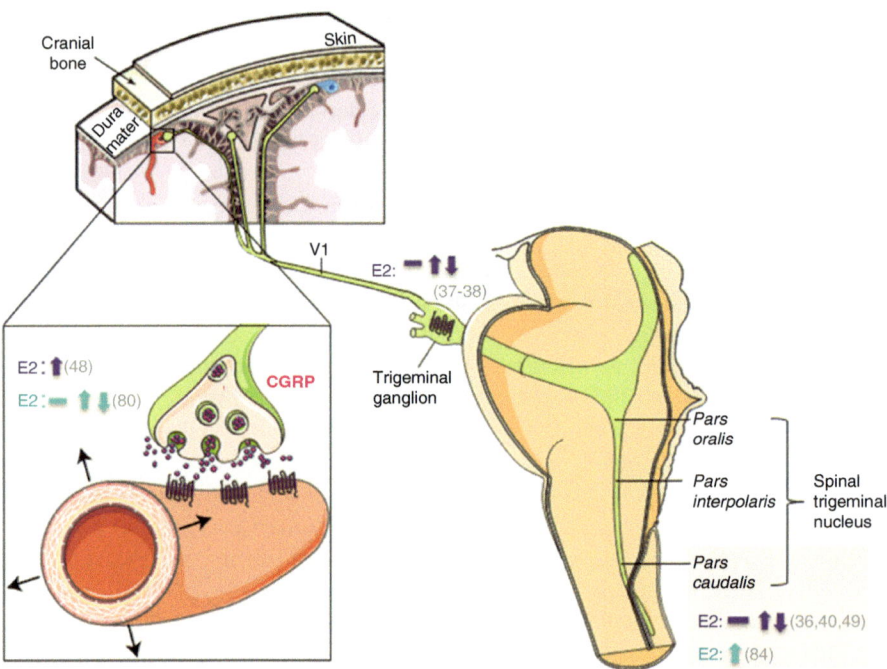

Fig. 7.1 The trigeminovascular system. Estradiol (E2) has been described to modify CGRP receptor expression and/or function in the peripheral and central components of the trigeminovascular system in rodents (purple) and humans (blue). Taken and modified from [56]

7.7   CGRP (Receptor) Blockade and Sex Differences

The acknowledgment of the role of CGRP in migraine led to the development of CGRP receptor antagonists (gepants) for the acute treatment of migraine attacks [85, 86]. One of them, telcagepant, was further evaluated for the treatment of peri-menstrual migraine and showed to be effective [87]. However, an increase in trans-aminases or pharmacokinetic restrictions was observed with gepants and all the clinical trials terminated [88, 89]. Currently, new gepants are under development.

The most recent approach for prophylactic migraine treatment are, in fact, four monoclonal antibodies against CGRP (eptinezumab, fremanezumab, and galcane-zumab) or its receptor (erenumab) [29–32]. No sex differences have been observed on the efficacy and tolerability of these antibodies; nevertheless, the precise mecha-nism of action has not been fully elucidated nor the possible side effects due to the long-term blockade of CGRP [90, 91]. Only fremanezumab was evaluated in a ran-domized double-blind, placebo-controlled study, where cardiovascular parameters in healthy perimenopausal women were assessed after the long-term blockade of CGRP and no hemodynamic changes were observed [92]. Considering the interaction between CGRP and ovarian steroid hormones, more studies should be performed to assess the cardiovascular safety in women.

7.8   Conclusions

The role of CGRP in migraine pathophysiology is clear. In view of the high female prevalence in migraine, it is evident that more studies should not only include females but should also investigate the relation between ovarian steroid hormones throughout the cycle and the CGRP pathway. Indeed, studies have already shown that CGRP expression and release are modulated by hormonal changes during the female cycle. Still, the exact mechanism has not been elucidated. More knowledge will not only contribute to a better understanding of the pathophysiology of migraine and the possible (side) effects of current therapies that block the CGRP pathway but may also lead to the development of novel, sex-specific antimigraine treatments.

References

1. Buse DC, Loder EW, Gorman JA, Stewart WF, Reed ML, Fanning KM, et al. Sex differences in the prevalence, symptoms, and associated features of migraine, probable migraine and other severe headache: results of the American Migraine Prevalence and Prevention (AMPP) study. Headache. 2013;53(8):1278–99.
2. Kurth T, Winter AC, Eliassen AH, Dushkes R, Mukamal KJ, Rimm EB, et al. Migraine and risk of cardiovascular disease in women: prospective cohort study. BMJ. 2016;353:i2610.
3. Somerville BW. The role of estradiol withdrawal in the etiology of menstrual migraine. Neurology. 1972;22(4):355.

4. Pavlović JM, Allshouse AA, Santoro NF, Crawford SL, Thurston RC, Neal-Perry GS, et al. Sex hormones in women with and without migraine. Evidence of migraine-specific hormone profiles. Neurology. 2016;87(1):49–56.
5. MacGregor EA, Frith A, Ellis J, Aspinall L, Hackshaw A. Incidence of migraine relative to menstrual cycle phases of rising and falling estrogen. Neurology. 2006;67(12):2154–8.
6. Somerville BW. The influence of progesterone and estradiol upon migraine. Headache: The Journal of Head and Face Pain. 1972;12(3):93–102.
7. Pringsheim T, Gooren L. Migraine prevalence in male to female transsexuals on hormone therapy. Neurology. 2004;63(3):593–4.
8. Martin VT, Pavlovic J, Fanning KM, Buse DC, Reed ML, Lipton RB. Perimenopause and menopause are associated with high frequency headache in women with migraine: results of the American Migraine Prevalence and Prevention study. Headache: The Journal of Head and Face Pain. 2016;56(2):292–305.
9. Kvisvik EV, Stovner LJ, Helde G, Bovim G, Linde M. Headache and migraine during pregnancy and puerperium: the MIGRA-study. J Headache Pain. 2011;12(4):443–51.
10. Glintborg D, Hass Rubin K, Nybo M, Abrahamsen B, Andersen M. Morbidity and medicine prescriptions in a nationwide Danish population of patients diagnosed with polycystic ovary syndrome. Eur J Endocrinol. 2015;172(5):627–38.
11. Tietjen GE, Conway A, Utley C, Gunning WT, Herial NA. Migraine is associated with menorrhagia and endometriosis. Headache: The Journal of Head and Face Pain. 2006;46(3):422–8.
12. Spierings ELH, Padamsee A. Menstrual-cycle and menstruation disorders in episodic vs chronic migraine: an exploratory study. Pain Med. 2015;16(7):1426–32.
13. Shuster LT, Faubion SS, Sood R, Casey PM. Hormonal manipulation strategies in the management of menstrual migraine and other hormonally related headaches. Curr Neurol Neurosci Rep. 2011;11(2):131–8.
14. Smitherman TA, Kolivas ED. Resolution of menstrually related migraine following aggressive treatment for breast cancer. Headache: The Journal of Head and Face Pain. 2010;50(3):485–8.
15. Goadsby PJ, Holland PR, Martins-Oliveira M, Hoffmann J, Schankin C, Akerman S. Pathophysiology of migraine: a disorder of sensory processing. Physiol Rev. 2017;97(2):553–622.
16. Edvinsson L. The trigeminovascular pathway: role of CGRP and CGRP receptors in migraine. Headache. 2017;57(Suppl 2):47–55.
17. Mayberg M, Langer RS, Zervas NT, Moskowitz MA. Perivascular meningeal projections from cat trigeminal ganglia: possible pathway for vascular headaches in man. Science. 1981;213(4504):228–30.
18. Goadsby PJ, Hoskin KL. The distribution of trigeminovascular afferents in the non-human primate brain Macaca nemestrina: a c-fos immunocytochemical study. J Anat. 1997;190(3):367–75.
19. Goadsby PJ, Lipton RB, Ferrari MD. Migraine — current understanding and treatment. N Engl J Med. 2002;346(4):257–70.
20. Russell FA, King R, Smillie SJ, Kodji X, Brain SD. Calcitonin gene-related peptide: physiology and pathophysiology. Physiol Rev. 2014;94(4):1099.
21. Amara SG, Jonas V, Rosenfeld MG, Ong ES, Evans RM. Alternative RNA processing in calcitonin gene expression generates mRNAs encoding different polypeptide products. Nature. 1982;298(5871):240–4.
22. Amara SG, Arriza JL, Leff SE, Swanson LW, Evans RM, Rosenfeld MG. Expression in brain of a messenger RNA encoding a novel neuropeptide homologous to calcitonin gene-related peptide. Science. 1985;229(4718):1094–7.
23. Eftekhari S, Salvatore CA, Johansson S, Chen TB, Zeng Z, Edvinsson L. Localization of CGRP, CGRP receptor, PACAP and glutamate in trigeminal ganglion. Relation to the blood-brain barrier. Brain Res. 2015;1600:93–109.
24. Eftekhari S, Warfvinge K, Blixt FW, Edvinsson L. Differentiation of nerve fibers storing CGRP and CGRP receptors in the peripheral trigeminovascular system. J Pain. 2013;14(11):1289–303.

25. Mulderry PK, Ghatei MA, Spokes RA, Jones PM, Pierson AM, Hamid QA, et al. Differential expression of alpha-CGRP and beta-CGRP by primary sensory neurons and enteric autonomic neurons of the rat. Neuroscience. 1988;25(1):195–205.
26. Goadsby PJ, Edvinsson L, Ekman R. Vasoactive peptide release in the extracerebral circulation of humans during migraine headache. Ann Neurol. 1990;28(2):183–7.
27. Goadsby PJ, Edvinsson L. The trigeminovascular system and migraine: studies characterizing cerebrovascular and neuropeptide changes seen in humans and cats. Ann Neurol. 1993;33(1):48–56.
28. Lassen LH, Haderslev PA, Jacobsen VB, Iversen HK, Sperling B, Olesen J. CGRP may play a causative role in migraine. Cephalalgia. 2002;22(1):54–61.
29. Silberstein SD, Dodick DW, Bigal ME, Yeung PP, Goadsby PJ, Blankenbiller T, et al. Fremanezumab for the preventive treatment of chronic migraine. N Engl J Med. 2017;377(22):2113–22.
30. Goadsby PJ, Reuter U, Hallström Y, Broessner G, Bonner JH, Zhang F, et al. A controlled trial of erenumab for episodic migraine. N Engl J Med. 2017;377(22):2123–32.
31. Skljarevski V, Oakes TM, Zhang Q, et al. Effect of different doses of galcanezumab vs placebo for episodic migraine prevention: a randomized clinical trial. JAMA Neurol. 2018;75:187.
32. Yuan H, Lauritsen CG, Kaiser EA, Silberstein SD. CGRP monoclonal antibodies for migraine: rationale and progress. BioDrugs. 2017;31(6):487–501.
33. Gupta S, McCarson KE, Welch KM, Berman NE. Mechanisms of pain modulation by sex hormones in migraine. Headache. 2011;51(6):905–22.
34. Bolay H, Berman NE, Akcali D. Sex-related differences in animal models of migraine headache. Headache. 2011;51(6):891–904.
35. Stucky NL, Gregory E, Winter MK, He YY, Hamilton ES, McCarson KE, et al. Sex differences in behavior and expression of CGRP-related genes in a rodent model of chronic migraine. Headache. 2011;51(5):674–92.
36. Vermeer LMM, Gregory E, Winter MK, McCarson KE, Berman NEJ. Exposure to bisphenol a exacerbates migraine-like behaviors in a multibehavior model of rat migraine. Toxicol Sci. 2014;137(2):416–27.
37. Giuffrè R, Palma E, Liccardo G, Sciarra F, Pastore F, Concolino G. Sex steroid hormones in the pathogenesis of chronic subdural haematoma. Neurochirurgia. 1992;35(04):103–7.
38. Gonzales RJ, Ansar S, Duckles SP, Krause DN. Androgenic/estrogenic balance in the male rat cerebral circulation: metabolic enzymes and sex steroid receptors. J Cereb Blood Flow Metab. 2007;27(11):1841–52.
39. Kemper MF, Zhao Y, Duckles SP, Krause DN. Endogenous ovarian hormones affect mitochondrial efficiency in cerebral endothelium via distinct regulation of PGC-1 isoforms. J Cereb Blood Flow Metab. 2013;33(1):122–8.
40. Zuloaga KL, O'Connor DT, Handa RJ, Gonzales RJ. Estrogen receptor beta dependent attenuation of cytokine-induced cyclooxygenase-2 by androgens in human brain vascular smooth muscle cells and rat mesenteric arteries. Steroids. 2012;77(8):835–44.
41. Puri V, Cui L, Liverman CS, Roby KF, Klein RM, Welch KMA, et al. Ovarian steroids regulate neuropeptides in the trigeminal ganglion. Neuropeptides. 2005;39(4):409–17.
42. Aggarwal M, Puri V, Puri S. Effects of estrogen on the serotonergic system and calcitonin gene-related peptide in trigeminal ganglia of rats. Ann Neurosci. 2012;19(4):151–7.
43. Bereiter DA, Cioffi JL, Bereiter DF. Oestrogen receptor-immunoreactive neurons in the trigeminal sensory system of male and cycling female rats. Arch Oral Biol. 2005;50(11):971–9.
44. Liverman C, Brown J, Sandhir R, McCarson K, Berman N. Role of the oestrogen receptors GPR30 and ERα in peripheral sensitization: relevance to trigeminal pain disorders in women. Cephalalgia. 2009;29(7):729–41.
45. Fenzi F, Rizzzuto N. Estrogen receptors localization in the spinal trigeminal nucleus: an immunohistochemical study in humans. Eur J Pain. 2011;15(10):1002–7.
46. Alimy-Allrath T, Ricken A, Bechmann I. Expression of estrogen receptors α and β in the trigeminal mesencephalic nucleus of adult women and men. Ann Anat. 2014;196(6):416–22.

47. Glinskii OV, Abraha TW, Turk JR, Rubin LJ, Huxley VH, Glinsky VV. Microvascular network remodeling in dura mater of ovariectomized pigs: role for angiopoietin-1 in estrogen-dependent control of vascular stability. Am J Physiol Heart Circ Physiol. 2007;293(2):H1131–H7.
48. Murata T, Dietrich HH, Xiang C, Dacey RG. G Protein–coupled estrogen receptor agonist improves cerebral microvascular function after hypoxia/reoxygenation injury in male and female rats. Stroke. 2013;44(3):779–85.
49. Meffre D, Delespierre B, Gouézou M, Leclerc P, Vinson GP, Schumacher M, et al. The membrane-associated progesterone-binding protein 25-Dx is expressed in brain regions involved in water homeostasis and is up-regulated after traumatic brain injury. J Neurochem. 2005;93(5):1314–26.
50. Khalid H, Shibata S, Kishikawa M, Yasunaga A, Iseki M, Hiura T. Immunohistochemical analysis of progesterone receptor and Ki-67 labeling index in astrocytic tumors. Cancer. 1997;80(11):2133.
51. Manteniotis S, Lehmann R, Flegel C, Vogel F, Hofreuter A, Schreiner BSP, et al. Comprehensive RNA-seq expression analysis of sensory ganglia with a focus on ion channels and GPCRs in trigeminal ganglia. PLoS One. 2013;8(11):e79523.
52. Haywood SA, Simonian SX, van der Beek EM, Bicknell RJ, Herbison AE. Fluctuating estrogen and progesterone receptor expression in brainstem norepinephrine neurons through the rat estrous cycle*. Endocrinology. 1999;140(7):3255–63.
53. Lin IC, Slemp AE, Hwang C, Karmacharya J, Gordon AD, Kirschner RE. Immunolocalization of androgen receptor in the developing craniofacial skeleton. J Craniofac Surg. 2004;15(6):922–7.
54. Lee KS, Zhang Y, Asgar J, Auh QS, Chung M-K, Ro JY. Androgen receptor transcriptionally regulates μ-opioid receptor expression in rat trigeminal ganglia. Neuroscience. 2016;331:52–61.
55. Simerly R, Swanson L, Chang C, Muramatsu M. Distribution of androgen and estrogen receptor mRNA-containing cells in the rat brain: an in situ hybridization study. J Comp Neurol. 1990;294(1):76–95.
56. Labastida-Ramirez A, Rubio-Beltran E, Villalon CM, MaassenVanDenBrink A. Gender aspects of CGRP in migraine. Cephalalgia. 2017.; 333102417739584.
57. Moussaoui S, Duval P, Lenoir V, Garret C, Kerdelhue B. CGRP in the trigeminal nucleus, spinal cord and hypothalamus: effect of gonadal steroids. Neuropeptides. 1996;30(6):546–50.
58. Wang D, Zhao J, Wang J, Li J, Yu S, Guo X. Deficiency of female sex hormones augments PGE2 and CGRP levels within midbrain periaqueductal gray. J Neurol Sci. 2014;346(1):107–11.
59. Pardutz A, Multon S, Malgrange B, Parducz A, Vecsei L, Schoenen J. Effect of systemic nitroglycerin on CGRP and 5-HT afferents to rat caudal spinal trigeminal nucleus and its modulation by estrogen. Eur J Neurosci. 2002;15(11):1803–9.
60. Gon G, Giaid A, Steel JH, O'Halloran DJ, Noorden SV, Ghatei MA, et al. Localization of immunoreactivity for calcitonin gene- related peptide in the rat anterior pituitary during ontogeny and gonadal steroid manipulations and detection of its messenger ribonucleic acid. Endocrinology. 1990;127(6):2618–29.
61. Yang Y, Ozawa H, Lu H, Yuri K, Hayashi S, Nihonyanagi K, et al. Immunocytochemical analysis of sex differences in calcitonin gene-related peptide in the rat dorsal root ganglion, with special reference to estrogen and its receptor. Brain Res. 1998;791(1):35–42.
62. Gangula PRR, Lanlua P, Wimalawansa S, Supowit S, DiPette D, Yallampalli C. Regulation of calcitonin gene-related peptide expression in dorsal root ganglia of rats by female sex steroid hormones1. Biol Reprod. 2000;62(4):1033–9.
63. Mowa CN, Usip S, Collins J, Storey-Workley M, Hargreaves KM, Papka RE. The effects of pregnancy and estrogen on the expression of calcitonin gene-related peptide (CGRP) in the uterine cervix, dorsal root ganglia and spinal cord. Peptides. 2003;24(8):1163–74.
64. Sarajari S, Oblinger MM. Estrogen effects on pain sensitivity and neuropeptide expression in rat sensory neurons. Exp Neurol. 2010;224(1):163–9.
65. Herbison AE, Spratt DP. Sexually dimorphic expression of calcitonin gene-related peptide (CGRP) mRNA in rat medial preoptic nucleus. Mol Brain Res. 1995;34(1):143–8.

66. Yuri K, Kawata M. Estrogen affects calcitonin gene-related peptide- and methionine-enkephalin-immunoreactive neuron in the female rat preoptic area. Neurosci Lett. 1994;169(1): 5–8.

67. Gupta S, Villalon CM, Mehrotra S, de Vries R, Garrelds IM, Saxena PR, et al. Female sex hormones and rat dural vasodilatation to CGRP, periarterial electrical stimulation and capsaicin. Headache. 2007;47(2):225–35.

68. Martin VT, Lee J, Behbehani MM. Sensitization of the trigeminal sensory system during different stages of the rat estrous cycle: implications for menstrual migraine. Headache. 2007;47(4):552–63.

69. Krause DN, Duckles SP, Pelligrino DA. Influence of sex steroid hormones on cerebrovascular function. J Appl Physiol. 2006;101(4):1252–61.

70. Jana B, Palus K, Meller K, Calka J. Porcine dorsal root ganglia ovarian neurons are affected by long lasting testosterone treatment. Physiol Res. 2016;65(6):1019–30.

71. Valdemarsson S, Edvinsson L, Hedner P, Ekman R. Hormonal influence on calcitonin gene-related peptide in man: effects of sex difference and contraceptive pills. Scand J Clin Lab Invest. 1990;50(4):385–8.

72. Ma QL, Zhou HY, Sun M. Relationship between sex hormone levels and blood calcitonin gene-related peptide/endothelin-1 in postmenopausal women with coronary heart disease. Hunan Yi Ke Da Xue Xue Bao. 2001;26(2):146–8.

73. Stevenson JC, Macdonald DW, Warren RC, Booker MW, Whitehead MI. Increased concentration of circulating calcitonin gene related peptide during normal human pregnancy. Br Med J (Clin Res Ed). 1986;293(6558):1329–30.

74. Caterina MJ, Schumacher MA, Tominaga M, Rosen TA, Levine JD, Julius D. The capsaicin receptor: a heat-activated ion channel in the pain pathway. Nature. 1997;389:816.

75. Van der Schueren BJ, Rogiers A, Vanmolkot FH, Van Hecken A, Depre M, Kane SA, et al. Calcitonin gene-related peptide8-37 antagonizes capsaicin-induced vasodilation in the skin: evaluation of a human in vivo pharmacodynamic model. J Pharmacol Exp Ther. 2008;325(1):248–55.

76. Sinclair SR, Kane SA, Van der Schueren BJ, Xiao A, Willson KJ, Boyle J, et al. Inhibition of capsaicin-induced increase in dermal blood flow by the oral CGRP receptor antagonist, telcagepant (MK-0974). Br J Clin Pharmacol. 2010;69(1):15–22.

77. Vermeersch S, Benschop RJ, Van Hecken A, Monteith D, Wroblewski VJ, Grayzel D, et al. Translational pharmacodynamics of calcitonin gene-related peptide monoclonal antibody LY2951742 in a capsaicin-induced dermal blood flow model. J Pharmacol Exp Ther. 2015;354(3):350–7.

78. Ibrahimi K, Vermeersch S, Frederiks P, Geldhof V, Draulans C, Buntinx L, et al. The influence of migraine and female hormones on capsaicin-induced dermal blood flow. Cephalalgia. 2017;37(12):1164–72.

79. Ibrahimi K, Vermeersch S, Danser A, Villalón C, Meiracker A, Hoon JD, et al. Development of an experimental model to study trigeminal nerve-mediated vasodilation on the human forehead. Cephalalgia. 2014;34(7):514–22.

80. Ibrahimi K, van Oosterhout WPJ, van Dorp W, Danser AHJ, Garrelds IM, Kushner SA, et al. Reduced trigeminovascular cyclicity in patients with menstrually related migraine. Neurology. 2015;84(2):125–31.

81. Gazerani P, Kaeseler Andersen O, Arendt-Nielsen L. A human experimental capsaicin model for trigeminal sensitization. Gender-specific differences. Pain. 2005;118(1):155–63.

82. Yamagata K, Sugimura M, Yoshida M, Sekine S, Kawano A, Oyamaguchi A, et al. Estrogens exacerbate nociceptive pain via up-regulation of TRPV1 and ANO1 in trigeminal primary neurons of female rats. Endocrinology. 2016;157(11):4309–17.

83. Schulte LH, May A. The migraine generator revisited: continuous scanning of the migraine cycle over 30 days and three spontaneous attacks. Brain. 2016;139(7):1987–93.

84. Maleki N, Linnman C, Brawn J, Burstein R, Becerra L, Borsook D. Her versus his migraine: multiple sex differences in brain function and structure. Brain. 2012;135(8):2546–59.

85. Ho TW, Mannix LK, Fan X, Assaid C, Furtek C, Jones CJ, et al. Randomized controlled trial of an oral CGRP receptor antagonist, MK-0974, in acute treatment of migraine. Neurology. 2008;70(16):1304–12.
86. Olesen J, Diener H-C, Husstedt IW, Goadsby PJ, Hall D, Meier U, et al. Calcitonin gene–related peptide receptor antagonist BIBN 4096 BS for the acute treatment of migraine. N Engl J Med. 2004;350(11):1104–10.
87. Ho TW, Ho A, Ge Y, Assaid C, Gottwald R, MacGregor EA, et al. Randomized controlled trial of the CGRP receptor antagonist telcagepant for prevention of headache in women with perimenstrual migraine. Cephalalgia. 2015;36(2):148–61.
88. Negro A, Lionetto L, Simmaco M, Martelletti P. CGRP receptor antagonists: an expanding drug class for acute migraine? Expert Opin Investig Drugs. 2012;21(6):807–18.
89. Ho TW, Connor KM, Zhang Y, Pearlman E, Koppenhaver J, Fan X, et al. Randomized controlled trial of the CGRP receptor antagonist telcagepant for migraine prevention. Neurology. 2014;83(11):958–66.
90. MaassenVanDenBrink A, Meijer J, Villalón CM, Ferrari MD. Wiping out CGRP: potential cardiovascular risks. Trends Pharmacol Sci. 2016;37(9):779–88.
91. Deen M, Correnti E, Kamm K, Kelderman T, Papetti L, Rubio-Beltran E, et al. Blocking CGRP in migraine patients - a review of pros and cons. J Headache Pain. 2017;18(1):96.
92. Bigal ME, Walter S, Bronson M, Alibhoy A, Escandon R. Cardiovascular and hemodynamic parameters in women following prolonged CGRP inhibition using LBR-101, a monoclonal antibody against CGRP. Cephalalgia. 2014;34(12):968–76.

Chapter 8
Gender Differences in Imaging Studies in Migraine

Nasim Maleki

Migraine is a common neurological disorder that is characterized by recurrent inter-mittent headaches (1–14 headache days per month in episodic migraine and >14 headache days in chronic migraine) that last 4–72 h. Migraine is considered by the World Health Organization (WHO) to be in the top 20 causes of disability world-wide [1] and affects patients during the most formative and productive periods of their lives. In the United States, migraine affects 30 million adults, and some 17% of American children have headaches including migraine [2] (Fig. 8.1).

Migraine also has a significant sex disparity in prevalence in adults with a higher prevalence in women [5] with an incidence rate that is about twice as high in women compared to men [6–8]. In children, however, this difference in prevalence does not exist during the prepubertal years with the incidence of migraine being similar in boys and girls during prepubertal phase [9]. A considerable number of boys become migraine-free once they reach puberty, while on the other hand, the migraine becomes more frequent or more intense in girls during that same period [10]. Moreover, there is a higher likelihood for girls to experience the onset of migraine in the same year that their menstrual periods start than any other time [11]. The mechanisms underlying the disease onset and evolution specifically the sex-specific shift in the pattern of disease incidence in puberty are unknown [12].

Evidence from various basic science, epidemiological, and clinical studies strongly suggests that ovarian steroids (that change substantially during puberty) have an important influence on the phenotypic expression of migraine [13–19]. In women especially, the ovarian steroid cycling has an impact on the biological mech-anisms of migraine. Changes in estrogen levels are thought to have an important influence on the phenotypic expression of migraine [11, 20, 21] in females: migraine can be triggered by the decline in estrogen that could occur naturally during the fall

N. Maleki (✉)
Psychiatric Neuroimaging Division, Department of Psychiatry, Massachusetts General Hospital, Harvard Medical School, Boston, MA, USA
e-mail: nmaleki@mgh.harvard.edu

© Springer Nature Switzerland AG 2019
A. Maassen van den Brink, E. A. MacGregor (eds.), *Gender and Migraine*, Headache, https://doi.org/10.1007/978-3-030-02988-3_8

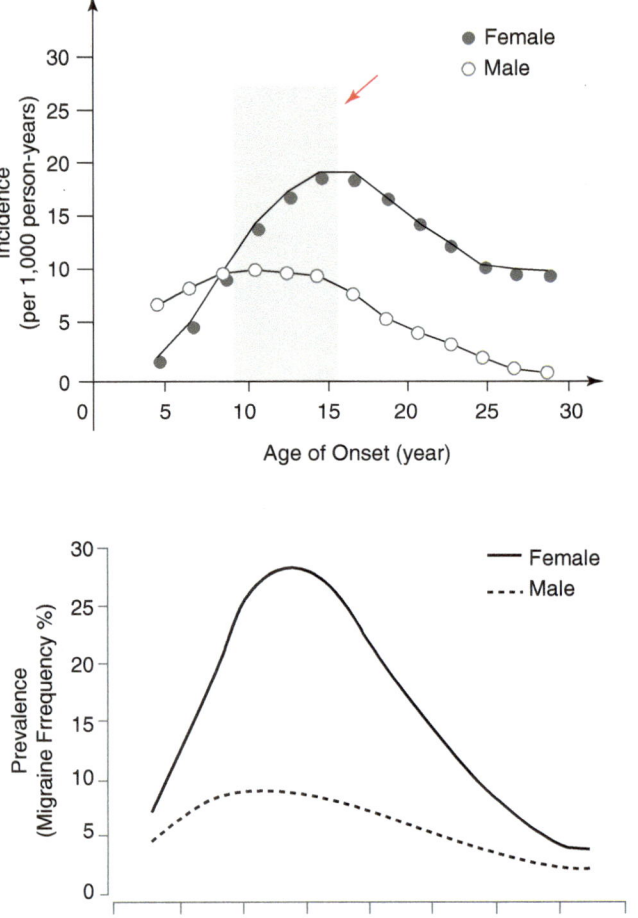

Fig. 8.1 Adjusted age-specific incidence (top) and prevalence (bottom) patterns of migraine by sex. Migraine is 2–3 times more prevalent in women. Sex-related differences in the incidence pattern start around puberty with a significantly higher incidence in girls compared to boys. Lipton and Bigal. Headache 2005. 45 Suppl 1: S3–S13. [3, 4]

in the estrogen immediately before menstruation and during the pill-free week in women who are on contraceptives or in women with bilateral oophorectomy [22].

There are changes in migraine patterns associated with menstrual periods, pregnancy, and menopause. Some women experience menstrual migraine or changes in the intensity or frequency of their migraine attacks during pregnancy. Migraine may improve during pregnancy, when estrogen levels rise gradually, but can reoccur immediately postpartum, when estrogen levels fall [11]. The hypothalamus secretes GnRH that signals the pituitary to secrete the reproductive hormones that influence menstruation. Sex steroids (such as estrogen) promote secondary sex characteristics in peripheral tissues and regulate GnRH neurons via negative neuro-endocrine feedback. These neurons originate in the nose and migrate into the brain, where they are scattered throughout the medial septum and hypothalamus [23].

The majority of women with migraine during the reproductive years become migraine-free after menopause. Moreover, it has been shown that in women, chronic migraine can be reversed to episodic migraine (in nearly 60% of individuals) by hormonal preventives [24]. Roughly 60% of women with migraine experience an attack pattern consistent with menstrually related migraine [13, 25]. Girls often experience the onset of migraine in the same year that their menstrual periods start [11] or their migraine becomes more frequent or more intense during that same period [10].

While the mechanisms of the migraine disease are still poorly understood, the sex-related epidemiological and clinical patterns described above have encouraged growing interest in examining sex differences in the brains of migraineurs as a way to better understand the pathophysiology of the disease. As advances in neuroimaging techniques have significantly improved our ability to assess the functional, morpho-metric, and chemical changes in the brain noninvasively, a growing number of neuroimaging studies have investigated the differences between the healthy brain and the migraine brain and have reported significant differences in multiple domains including the functional activity and connectivity, structural morphometry (thinning, thickening, volume increase or decrease), structural connectivity, and neurotransmitter or metabolite levels in the brain of migraine patients [26–33]. However, the sex specificity of such abnormalities and their links to the sex-related epidemiological and clinical patterns have been less studied and examined only in a limited number of studies.

In a study on sex-related differences in the structure and function of the brain of episodic migraine patients [34], two groups of opposite sex, age-matched migraine patients along with age- and sex-matched healthy control subjects, were recruited ($N = 11$ in each group). The patients in this study had all suffered from migraine for 3 years or longer and were matched for a number of attributes related to their migraine such as age of onset, medication type, and the average number of migraine attacks they experienced per month. The participants underwent high-resolution structural imaging as well as functional magnetic resonance imaging of the brain. High-resolution images of the brain were used to assess the thickness of the gray matter of the brain at a sub-millimeter level. Functional images of the brain were collected during evoked response to painful heat applied to the back of the hand. This study revealed:

1. Increased gray matter thickness in two areas of the brain that were specific only to women with migraine. These areas included the insula, which is an area in the brain involved in processing pain, interoception [35], autonomic function [36, 37], sensation [38, 39], and affective processing, and the precuneus that is less known to do with pain processing but more with self-awareness.

2. Reduction of the volume of the parahippocampal gyrus in male migraineurs. The parahippocampal gyrus surrounds the hippocampus and is involved in numerous behaviors including stress and anxiety.
3. More pronounced brain response to pain in women with migraine in brain regions involved in emotional processing such as the amygdala which was consistent with increased measures of pain unpleasantness for these women too (Fig. 8.2).

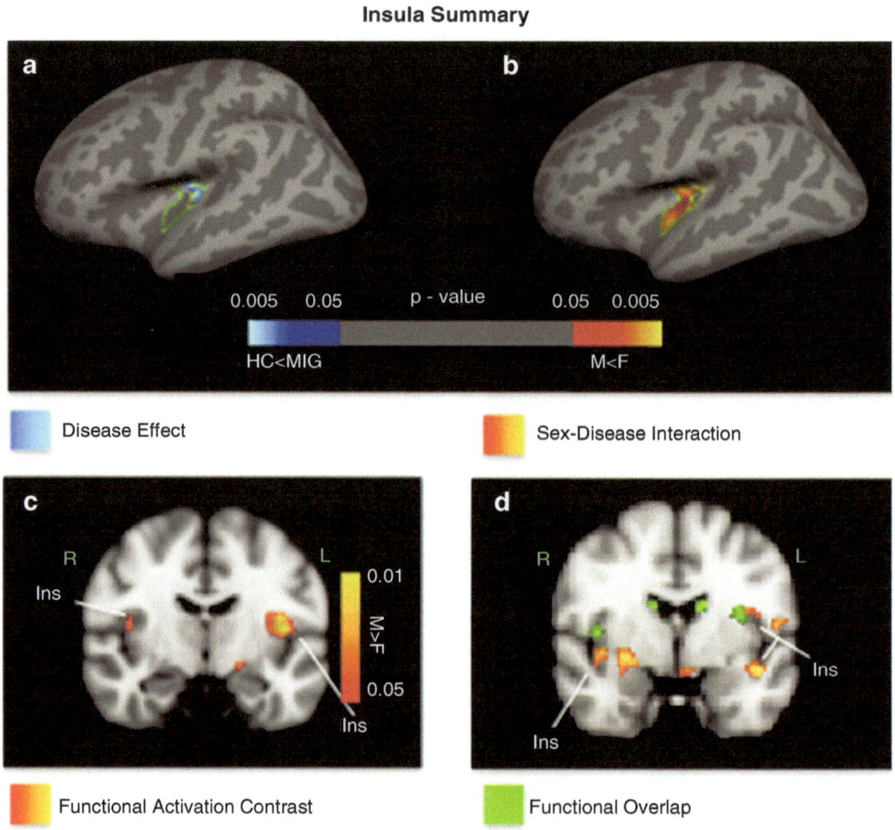

Fig. 8.2 Sex-related structural and functional insular abnormalities. Results of the comparisons conducted on female (F) vs. male (M) migraine patients versus healthy control subjects are shown. First row: (**a**) the disease effects on cortical thickness (blue-light blue) and (**b**) sex-disease interaction (red-yellow) are shown for the insula that is thicker in female migraineurs relative to healthy female subjects and also relative to both healthy and migraineur male subjects. Bottom row: (**c**) functional activation contrast map (male < female) in response to painful heat stimulation shows significant difference in insular activity in male versus female migraineurs and (**d**) overlap of disease-related functional differences between female migraineurs vs. female healthy control subjects (in green) and sex-related differences in female vs. male migraineurs in response to painful stimulation overlap in insula. Adapted from Maleki et al. [34]

A follow-up study evaluated changes in the cortical thickness by age in 92 female subjects (46 patients with migraine and 46 healthy controls) using high-field magnetic resonance imaging [40]. An abnormal pattern of bilateral lack of thinning of gray matter in the insula of adult female migraineurs was observed. While this was a cross-sectional study, the observed pattern was in contrast to the patterns of insular thinning reported in cross-sectional studies of healthy subjects where the relative gray matter loss rate of the insular cortex is reported approximately double of that seen in other cortical areas during aging [41]. Insular abnormalities in association with migraine are also reported in a number of other neuroimaging studies [32, 42–45].

A number of neuroimaging studies have assessed sex-related differences in the brain's intrinsic functional connectivity. In this approach, functional networks are derived from estimating correlations between time courses of brain activity in different regions which allows determining networks of functionally connected structures in the absence of an active task or an experimental manipulation. In one study, resting-state brain functional networks were compared in 38 migraine patients (20 females) and 38 healthy subjects (20 females). Using graph theory analysis, network properties such as small-worldness, network resilience, nodal centrality, and interregional connections were compared between these groups. The study revealed that there were more alterations of topological properties present in the brain functional networks of female migraineurs with more regions in the female migraineurs showing decreased nodal centrality (index for evaluating the importance of nodes within functional networks) and worse resilience which may reflect faulty communication within and between brain regions in female migraineurs. One of the main resting-state brain functional networks is the default mode network (DMN) [46] that is a neural network that is the most active at rest but deactivated when the brain is actively involved in external attention demanding goal-directed tasks. Default mode network includes precuneus, posterior cingulate, medial prefrontal, medial temporal lobe, and angular gyrus [47]. While the influence of hormonal fluctuations on the dysfunctional organization of RSNs in women with migraine needs to yet be studied, other studies in healthy women have shown that the resting-state functional intrinsic connectivity between the DMN and the executive control network (ECN) is modulated by the phase of the menstrual cycle (i.e., follicular vs. luteal) and also by the usage of oral contraceptive pills especially in the anterior cingulate cortex [48].

A more recent neuroimaging study [49] also using graph theory and a precise parcellation atlas of the brain (Brainnetome atlas [50]) to examine the topological organization of the functional networks of resting-state brain functional networks in 29 female migraineurs without aura and 29 female age-matched healthy controls has further revealed widespread disrupted functional connectivity in female migraineurs. In particular, the posterior insula exhibited decreased nodal centrality, smaller volume, and disrupted connectivity with many other brain areas in female migraineurs compared to healthy women. The study showed that the disrupted connections primarily involved subregions of the brain involved in the discrimination of sensory features of pain, pain modulation or processing, and sensory integration processing (Fig. 8.3).

These studies suggest that functional networks of the female brain may be more vulnerable to dysfunctional organization [51]. This notion is further supported by another recent analysis of resting-state connectivity in 29 women with chronic migraine compared to 19 age- and sex-matched controls [52]. The findings revealed significant decrease in the resting functional connectivity of three major intrinsic brain networks in women with chronic migraine. These networks include the default mode network, salience network, and central executive network. Reduced connectivity in salience and executive networks was also associated with higher frequency of migraine attacks in these patients.

There are also sex-related differences in the incidence of brain white matter abnormalities in migraine patients. These abnormalities, which appear as small regions of high intensity on MRI images, are more prevalent in migraineurs than the general population [53]. Among women, deep white matter hyperintensity volume as well as the incidence of progression is greater in migraineurs than their matched healthy controls [53] which may reflect potential differences in the inflammatory markers in female vs. male migraineurs or, alternatively, sex differences in the sensitivity or the brain region-specific expression of the inflammatory marker receptors in the brain of female migraineurs or the modulatory effect of hormones on the inflammatory markers.

Finally, most recent advances in the field of migraine research have provided strong evidence for a link between the hypothalamus and migraine [54]. Research has suggested a main central role for the hypothalamus and its ascending and descending connections to pain-processing structures in the brain in the pathophysiology of migraine [42, 55] and the premonitory symptoms of a migraine attack that are mainly of hypothalamic origin. Recent positron emission tomography (PET)

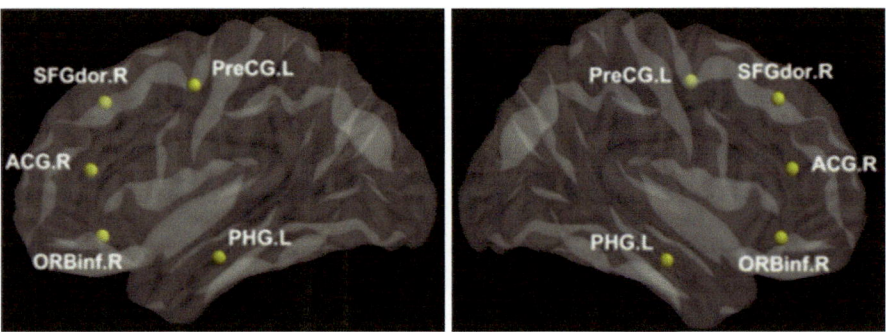

Fig. 8.3 Significant sex-related resting network differences. Comparing the brain's resting functional networks between migraineurs and healthy subjects revealed prominent nodal centrality differences in the precentral gyrus (PreCG), dorsolateral superior frontal gyrus (SFGdor), orbital inferior frontal gyrus (ORBinf), anterior cingulate gyrus (ACG), and parahippocampal gyrus (PHG) that showed interaction between sex (male vs. female) and disease state (patients vs. controls). Adapted from Liu et al. [51]

studies on patients during a migraine attack have further emphasized a pivotal role for hypothalamus in migraine onset and pathology [42, 55]. The hypothalamus is involved in the maintenance of the homeostasis in the body that is mediated by autonomic system signaling and through endocrine signals to the hypothalamus–pituitary–gonadal (HPG) and the hypothalamus–pituitary–adrenal axis. Given that the hypothalamus is part of the HPG axis, which is a central control and regulatory system that connects the central nervous system (CNS) with the reproductive hormonal system, and the important role that the ovarian steroid cycling has on the biological mechanisms of migraine, it is likely that some sex-related differences in migraine may have hypothalamic origin. Although this link has to be yet determined through more studies, there may be sex-related differences in hormonal abnormalities or in their modulatory effects on brain activity. For instance, a recent study of 119 migraine patients [56] showed that male migraineurs have lower progesterone levels compared to healthy males, whereas female migraineurs have lower follicular phase testosterone levels and lower luteal phase estrogen and testosterone levels compared to healthy females. Higher prevalence of depression and anxiety [57, 58] in female migraineurs may further implicate a role for hypothalamus in mediating sex-related differences in migraine.

There are multiple unmet needs in neuroimaging study of sex-related differences in migraine. To date, all of the studies on sex-related differences in migraine been have been done interictally and have focused on abnormalities in the brain outside of an attack; studies during the ictal phase with a naturally occurring or an invoked attack are still lacking. Moreover, all studies to date have relied on blood oxygenation level-dependent (BOLD) functional magnetic resonance imaging (fMRI) to study the functional activity and connectivity of the migraine brain. BOLD-fMRI is a hemodynamic-based approach that, because of the coupling between the neuronal activity and the changes in the blood flow, can serve as a proxy for functional activity. However, functional activity in the brain is associated with electromagnetic and metabolic changes, in addition to hemodynamic changes. Therefore, while BOLD-fMRI is a strong technique, it lacks the excellent temporal resolution of the methods that rely on changes in the electrical potentials and magnetic field in the brain such as electroencephalography (EEG) and magnetoencephalography (MEG). Incorporating EEG and MEG in assessing sex-related differences may reveal additional insights into the pathophysiology of the disease. There are other unexplored neuroimaging areas in studying the sex-related differences in migraine such as magnetic resonance spectroscopy or positron emission tomography that are sensitive to metabolic changes with the latter also allowing tracking of various distinctively labeled cell types or receptors. For instance, using magnetic resonance spectroscopy on a high-power scanner (7 T), a recent study [59] has revealed higher glutamate levels in the visual cortex of migraine patients without aura providing more evidence for a pathophysiological link between glutamate and migraine via its neuro-excitatory effects, or its role in energy metabolism, or both.

Finally, it should be noted that one major limitation in neuroimaging studies in migraine is that female patients have dominated the majority of studies and there is a need for more studies in men. This is particularly important because basic science studies mostly solely include male animals. Overall, in order to allow a better translation between basic science research and studies in human, particularly neuroimaging studies in humans, paying attention to sex-related differences in both the design and interpretation of the findings is a must. Indeed, neuroimaging studies on sex-related differences in migraine seem to confirm differences in the brains of men and women who suffer from migraine. The differences seem to involve both the structure of the brain and the functional activity and connectivity of the brain.

References

1. Buse DC, Rupnow MF, Lipton RB. Assessing and managing all aspects of migraine: migraine attacks, migraine-related functional impairment, common comorbidities, and quality of life. Mayo Clin Proc. 2009;84(5):422–35. https://doi.org/10.4065/84.5.422. 84/5/422 [pii].
2. Lateef TM, Merikangas KR, He J, Kalaydjian A, Khoromi S, Knight E, Nelson KB. Headache in a national sample of American children: prevalence and comorbidity. J Child Neurol. 2009;24(5):536–43. https://doi.org/10.1177/0883073808327831. 24/5/536 [pii].
3. Lipton RB, Stewart WF, Diamond S, Diamond ML, Reed M. Prevalence and burden of migraine in the United States: data from the American Migraine Study II. Headache 2001; 41(7):646–57. PMID: 11554952.
4. Stewart WF, Linet MS, Celentano DD, Van Natta M, Ziegler D. Age- and sex-specific incidence rates of migraine with and without visual aura. Am J Epidemiol 1991;134(10):1111–20. PMID: 1746521.
5. Stewart WF, Lipton RB, Celentano DD, Reed ML. Prevalence of migraine headache in the United States. Relation to age, income, race, and other sociodemographic factors. JAMA. 1992;267(1):64–9.
6. Brandes JL. The influence of estrogen on migraine: a systematic review. JAMA. 2006;295(15):1824–30.
7. Le H, Tfelt-Hansen P, Russell MB, Skytthe A, Kyvik KO, Olesen J. Co-morbidity of migraine with somatic disease in a large population-based study. Cephalalgia. 2011;31(1):43–64. https://doi.org/10.1177/0333102410373159.
8. Russell MB, Rasmussen BK, Thorvaldsen P, Olesen J. Prevalence and sex-ratio of the subtypes of migraine. Int J Epidemiol. 1995;24(3):612–8.
9. Pakalnis A, Gladstein J. Headaches and hormones. Semin Pediatr Neurol. 2010;17(2):100–4. https://doi.org/10.1016/j.spen.2010.04.007. S1071-9091(10)00036-7 [pii].
10. Russell MB, Rasmussen BK, Fenger K, Olesen J. Migraine without aura and migraine with aura are distinct clinical entities: a study of four hundred and eighty-four male and female migraineurs from the general population. Cephalalgia. 1996;16(4):239–45.
11. Silberstein SD, Lipton RB, Dodick D, Wolff HG. Wolff's headache and other head pain. 8th ed. Oxford; New York, NY: Oxford University Press; 2008.
12. Greenspan JD, Craft RM, LeResche L, Arendt-Nielsen L, Berkley KJ, Fillingim RB, et al. Studying sex and gender differences in pain and analgesia: a consensus report. Pain. 2007;132(Suppl 1):S26–45.
13. Epstein MT, Hockaday JM, Hockaday TD. Migraine and reproductive hormones throughout the menstrual cycle. Lancet. 1975;1(7906):543–8.
14. Goldstein M, Chen TC. The epidemiology of disabling headache. Adv Neurol. 1982;33: 377–90.
15. Lipton RB, Stewart WF. Migraine in the United States: a review of epidemiology and health care use. Neurology. 1993;43(6 Suppl 3):S6–10.
16. Silberstein SD. Sex hormones and headache. Rev Neurol. 2000;156(Suppl 4):4S30–41.

17. Silberstein SD, Merriam GR. Estrogens, progestins, and headache. Neurology. 1991;41(6):786–93.
18. Silberstein SD, Merriam GR. Physiology of the menstrual cycle. Cephalalgia. 2000;20(3):148–54.
19. Silberstein S, Merriam G. Sex hormones and headache 1999 (menstrual migraine). Neurology. 1999;53(4 Suppl 1):S3–13.
20. Martin VT. New theories in the pathogenesis of menstrual migraine. Curr Pain Headache Rep. 2008;12(6):453–62.
21. Martin VT, Behbehani M. Ovarian hormones and migraine headache: understanding mechanisms and pathogenesis--part I. Headache. 2006;46(1):3–23. https://doi.org/10.1111/j.1526-4610.2006.00309.x.
22. Sacco S, Ricci S, Degan D, Carolei A. Migraine in women: the role of hormones and their impact on vascular diseases. J Headache Pain. 2012;13(3):177–89. https://doi.org/10.1007/s10194-012-0424-y.
23. Sisk CL, Zehr JL. Pubertal hormones organize the adolescent brain and behavior. Front Neuroendocrinol. 2005;26(3-4):163–74. https://doi.org/10.1016/j.yfrne.2005.10.003.
24. Calhoun A, Ford S. Elimination of menstrual-related migraine beneficially impacts chronification and medication overuse. Headache. 2008;48(8):1186–93.
25. Loder G, Silberstein S. Headaches in women. In: Wolff's headache. 8th ed. New York, NY: Oxford University Press; 2008. p. 691–710.
26. Burstein R, Jakubowski M, Garcia-Nicas E, Kainz V, Bajwa Z, Hargreaves R, et al. Thalamic sensitization transforms localized pain into widespread allodynia. Ann Neurol. 2010;68(1):81–91. https://doi.org/10.1002/ana.21994.
27. Mailis-Gagnon A, Giannoylis I, Downar J, Kwan CL, Mikulis DJ, Crawley AP, et al. Altered central somatosensory processing in chronic pain patients with "hysterical" anesthesia. Neurology. 2003;60(9):1501–7.
28. Maleki N, Becerra L, Brawn J, Bigal M, Burstein R, Borsook D. Concurrent functional and structural cortical alterations in migraine. Cephalalgia. 2012a;32(8):607–20. https://doi.org/10.1177/0333102412445622.
29. Maleki N, Becerra L, Upadhyay J, Burstein R, Borsook D. Direct optic nerve pulvinar connections defined by diffusion MR tractography in humans: implications for photophobia. Hum Brain Mapp. 2012b;33(1):75–88. https://doi.org/10.1002/hbm.21194.
30. Moulton EA, Burstein R, Tully S, Hargreaves R, Becerra L, Borsook D. Interictal dysfunction of a brainstem descending modulatory center in migraine patients. PLoS One. 2008;3(11):e3799. https://doi.org/10.1371/journal.pone.0003799.
31. Russo A, Tessitore A, Esposito F, Marcuccio L, Giordano A, Conforti R, et al. Pain processing in patients with migraine: an event-related fMRI study during trigeminal nociceptive stimulation. J Neurol. 2012;259:1903–12. https://doi.org/10.1007/s00415-012-6438-1.
32. Schmidt-Wilcke T, Ganssbauer S, Neuner T, Bogdahn U, May A. Subtle grey matter changes between migraine patients and healthy controls. Cephalalgia. 2008;28(1):1–4. https://doi.org/10.1111/j.1468-2982.2007.01428.x.
33. Tessitore A, Russo A, Esposito F, Giordano A, Taglialatela G, De Micco R, et al. Interictal cortical reorganization in episodic migraine without aura: an event-related fMRI study during parametric trigeminal nociceptive stimulation. Neurol Sci. 2011;32(Suppl 1):S165–7. https://doi.org/10.1007/s10072-011-0537-0.
34. Maleki N, Linnman C, Brawn J, Burstein R, Becerra L, Borsook D. Her versus his migraine: multiple sex differences in brain function and structure. Brain. 2012c;135(Pt 8):2546–59. https://doi.org/10.1093/brain/aws175.
35. Craig AD. How do you feel--now? The anterior insula and human awareness. Nat Rev Neurosci. 2009;10(1):59–70. https://doi.org/10.1038/nrn2555.
36. Beissner F, Meissner K, Bar KJ, Napadow V. The autonomic brain: an activation likelihood estimation meta-analysis for central processing of autonomic function. J Neurosci. 2013;33(25):10503–11. https://doi.org/10.1523/JNEUROSCI.1103-13.2013.

37. Critchley HD, Nagai Y, Gray MA, Mathias CJ. Dissecting axes of autonomic control in humans: insights from neuroimaging. Auton Neurosci. 2011;161(1-2):34–42. https://doi.org/10.1016/j.autneu.2010.09.005.
38. Henderson LA, Gandevia SC, Macefield VG. Somatotopic organization of the processing of muscle and cutaneous pain in the left and right insula cortex: a single-trial fMRI study. Pain. 2007;128(1-2):20–30. https://doi.org/10.1016/j.pain.2006.08.013.
39. Nieuwenhuys R. The insular cortex: a review. Prog Brain Res. 2012;195:123–63. https://doi.org/10.1016/B978-0-444-53860-4.00007-6.
40. Maleki N, Barmettler G, Moulton EA, Scrivani S, Veggeberg R, Spierings EL, et al. Female migraineurs show lack of insular thinning with age. Pain. 2015;156(7):1232–9. https://doi.org/10.1097/j.pain.0000000000000159.
41. Grieve SM, Clark CR, Williams LM, Peduto AJ, Gordon E. Preservation of limbic and paralimbic structures in aging. Hum Brain Mapp. 2005;25(4):391–401. https://doi.org/10.1002/hbm.20115.
42. Bahra A, Matharu MS, Buchel C, Frackowiak RS, Goadsby PJ. Brainstem activation specific to migraine headache. Lancet. 2001;357(9261):1016–7.
43. Kim JH, Kim S, Suh SI, Koh SB, Park KW, Oh K. Interictal metabolic changes in episodic migraine: a voxel-based FDG-PET study. Cephalalgia. 2010;30(1):53–61. https://doi.org/10.1111/j.1468-2982.2009.01890.x.
44. Xue T, Yuan K, Zhao L, Yu D, Zhao L, Dong T, et al. Intrinsic brain network abnormalities in migraines without aura revealed in resting-state fMRI. PLoS One. 2012;7(12):e52927. https://doi.org/10.1371/journal.pone.0052927.
45. Yang J, Zeng F, Feng Y, Fang L, Qin W, Liu X, et al. A PET-CT study on the specificity of acupoints through acupuncture treatment in migraine patients. BMC Complement Altern Med. 2012;12:123. https://doi.org/10.1186/1472-6882-12-123.
46. Raichle ME, Snyder AZ. A default mode of brain function: a brief history of an evolving idea. Neuroimage. 2007;37(4):1083–90. https://doi.org/10.1016/j.neuroimage.2007.02.041. discussion 1097–1089.
47. Buckner RL, Andrews-Hanna JR, Schacter DL. The brain's default network: anatomy, function, and relevance to disease. Ann N Y Acad Sci. 2008;1124:1–38. https://doi.org/10.1196/annals.1440.011.
48. Petersen N, Kilpatrick LA, Goharzad A, Cahill L. Oral contraceptive pill use and menstrual cycle phase are associated with altered resting state functional connectivity. Neuroimage. 2014;90:24–32. https://doi.org/10.1016/j.neuroimage.2013.12.016.
49. Zhang J, Su J, Wang M, Zhao Y, Zhang QT, Yao Q, et al. The posterior insula shows disrupted brain functional connectivity in female migraineurs without aura based on brainnetome atlas. Sci Rep. 2017;7(1):16868. https://doi.org/10.1038/s41598-017-17069-8.
50. Fan L, Li H, Zhuo J, Zhang Y, Wang J, Chen L, et al. The human Brainnetome Atlas: a new brain atlas based on connectional architecture. Cereb Cortex. 2016;26(8):3508–26. https://doi.org/10.1093/cercor/bhw157.
51. Liu J, Qin W, Nan J, Li J, Yuan K, Zhao L, et al. Gender-related differences in the dysfunctional resting networks of migraine suffers. PLoS One. 2011;6(11):e27049. https://doi.org/10.1371/journal.pone.0027049.
52. Androulakis XM, Krebs K, Peterlin BL, Zhang T, Maleki N, Sen S, et al. Modulation of intrinsic resting-state fMRI networks in women with chronic migraine. Neurology. 2017;89(2):163–9. https://doi.org/10.1212/WNL.0000000000004089.
53. Kruit MC, van Buchem MA, Launer LJ, Terwindt GM, Ferrari MD. Migraine is associated with an increased risk of deep white matter lesions, subclinical posterior circulation infarcts and brain iron accumulation: the population-based MRI CAMERA study. Cephalalgia. 2010;30(2):129–36. https://doi.org/10.1111/j.1468-2982.2009.01904.x. CHA1904 [pii].
54. Maniyar FH, Sprenger T, Monteith T, Schankin C, Goadsby PJ. Brain activations in the premonitory phase of nitroglycerin-triggered migraine attacks. Brain. 2013; https://doi.org/10.1093/brain/awt320.

55. Afridi SK, Matharu MS, Lee L, Kaube H, Friston KJ, Frackowiak RS, Goadsby PJ. A PET study exploring the laterality of brainstem activation in migraine using glyceryl trinitrate. Brain. 2005;128(Pt 4):932–9. https://doi.org/10.1093/brain/awh416.
56. Li W, Diao X, Chen C, Li C, Zhang Y, Li Y. Changes in hormones of the hypothalamic-pituitary-gonadal axis in migraine patients. J Clin Neurosci. 2018; https://doi.org/10.1016/j.jocn.2017.11.011.
57. Guidetti V, Alberton S, Galli F, Salvi E. Gender, migraine and affective disorders in the course of the life cycle. Funct Neurol. 2009;24(1):29–40. 3374 [pii].
58. Hedborg K, Anderberg UM, Muhr C. Stress in migraine: personality-dependent vulnerability, life events, and gender are of significance. Ups J Med Sci. 2011;116(3):187–99. https://doi.org/10.3109/03009734.2011.573883.
59. Zielman R, Wijnen JP, Webb A, Onderwater GLJ, Ronen I, Ferrari MD, et al. Cortical gluta-mate in migraine. Brain. 2017;140(7):1859–71. https://doi.org/10.1093/brain/awx130.

Chapter 9
Transgender and Migraine

E. Anne MacGregor and Antoinette Maassen van den Brink

9.1 Introduction

The term 'transgender' refers to people whose sex they were assigned at birth differs from the one they identify with. It is one of the categories of several gender identities that refer to an individual's self-identification as a man or woman, or occasionally undefined, as listed in Table 9.1.

Although recognised throughout history, it was not until the twentieth century when it was formalised and the term 'transsexual' was first used. Transsexuality was

Table 9.1 Definitions [1]

Gender identity	A person's internal sense of gender, usually binary (male or female)
Transgender	People whose gender is different from their sex designated at birth, usually shortened to 'trans'
Transgender man	Assigned female at birth but identifies as a man and may have had cross-sex hormone therapy or sex reassignment surgery (SRS) or both
Transgender woman	Assigned male at birth but identifies as a woman and may have had cross-sex hormone therapy or sex reassignment surgery (SRS) or both
Transsexual	A historical term, still in occasional use, to describe people who have permanently transitioned to their identified gender
Non-binary	People who identify as neither male nor female
Cisgender	People who are not transgender

E. A. MacGregor (✉)
Barts Health NHS Trust, London, UK
e-mail: anne@annemacgregor.com

A. Maassen van den Brink
Division of Vascular Medicine and Pharmacology, Department of Internal Medicine, Erasmus University Medical Center, Rotterdam, The Netherlands
e-mail: a.vanharen-maassenvandenbrink@erasmusmc.nl

© Springer Nature Switzerland AG 2019   113
A. Maassen van den Brink, E. A. MacGregor (eds.), *Gender and Migraine*,
Headache, https://doi.org/10.1007/978-3-030-02988-3_9

first included in the *Diagnostic and Statistical Manual of Mental Disorders, Third Edition (DSM-3)*. A mismatch between sex designated at birth and an individual's gender identity can be associated with significant stress when unrecognised or untreated and so is diagnosed as 'gender dysphoria' in the *DSM-5*, which replaces the *DSM-4* term 'gender identity disorder' [2]. This was in recognition that distress was the relevant parameter and a mismatch itself should not be considered pathological. The term transgender is now more commonly used than transsexual, although the latter term remains in the *International Statistical Classification of Diseases and Related Health Problems, Tenth Edition (ICD-10)*. However, there is pressure to remove this category in the *ICD-11*.

The aim of this review is to focus specifically on the issues relating to migraine and its management in transgender men and women.

9.2   Manifestations

Transgender is considered to be the consequence of highly complex genetic, neurodevelopmental and psychological factors and can include the desire to be of an alternative gender, not just binary.

The manifestations of transgender vary according to age group. Prepubertal children will show a clear preference to dress and play like their opposite sex, which can result in significant distress if pressured to behave otherwise. They may express dislike of their primary sex characteristics. With the onset of puberty, adolescents become increasingly concerned about the development of secondary sex characteristics that they do not identify with. Transgender adults adopt the dress and behaviour of their preferred gender and integrate socially as such. Both adolescents and adults may seek either hormonal treatment or surgery or both.

9.3   Prevalence

Prevalence depends on the definition of transgender used. A systematic review of 27 studies reported an overall meta-prevalence estimate of 355 per 100,000 population (0.355%) [3]. Other studies suggest a higher prevalence ranging from 0.5% to 1.3% for birth-assigned males and from 0.4% to 1.2% for birth-assigned females [4]. Based on the lower estimate of 0.5%, this equates to around 25 million transgender people worldwide.

With increasing destigmatisation of being transgender, prevalence rates are likely to increase significantly in all age groups. At the Tavistock Gender Identity Development Service in London, UK, overall referral rates doubled in the year 2015/2016 and continue to rise. Until recently, the majority of referral was for birthassigned boys, reflecting the greater number of adult transgender women compared to transgender men. This is now changing, and the referral rate of birth-assigned

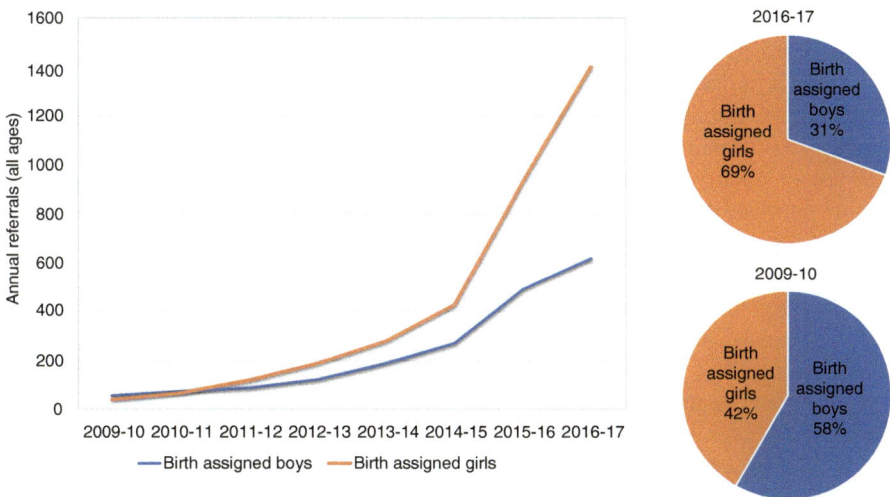

Fig. 9.1 Referral rates of birth-assigned boys and girls to the Gender Identity Development Service at the Tavistock Centre, London, UK [5]

girls overtook birth-assigned boys for the first time in the year 2010/2011, with over 70% of referrals in 2016 being birth-assigned girls (Fig. 9.1) [5].

According to *DSM-5*, the prevalence of gender dysphoria is 0.005–0.014% for adult birth-assigned males and 0.002–0.003% for adult birth-assigned females [2]. In children, gender dysphoria has been 2–4.5 times more common among birth-assigned boys than among birth-assigned girls, while in adolescents, the male-to-female ratio has been closer to parity [2]. However, as referral rates increase, the prevalence of gender dysphoria is likely to increase accordingly particularly in the absence of access to specialist services.

9.4 Relevance to Migraine

Significant sex differences exist in migraine, which is known to affect three times more women than men, particularly during the reproductive years [6]. The difference is considered to be due to the additional effects of oestrogen in women, with falling levels associated with migraine without aura and high levels associated with migraine aura [7].

While it is to be expected that hormone therapy will affect migraine in transgender people, the data are extremely limited. A Dutch questionnaire survey found a migraine prevalence of 26% in transgender women who had recently completed sex reassignment surgery and who used anti-androgens to suppress male sex characteristics together with oestrogens to induce female sex characteristics [8]. This prevalence is similar to the migraine prevalence of 25% in cisgender women in the same population and significantly higher than the reported prevalence of 7.5% in cisgender men [9]. Prevalence of visual aura was also higher than expected, reported by 54%, again supporting the effect of high oestrogen states on migraine aura [8].

There are no prevalence data for migraine before and after hormone therapy, but an Italian study of pain in 47 transgender women found an increase in headache following the use of feminising hormones: of 47 transgender women, two reported headache before hormone therapy, increasing to five reporting headache following treatment [10].

The same study suggests that testosterone therapy can benefit headache: of 26 transgender men, ten reported headache before hormone therapy, 6 reported a reduction in frequency and severity of headache following treatment and three reported onset of headache [10].

These findings are important for management and highlight the need for clinicians to consider the effects of hormone treatment on migraine and advise transgender patients accordingly. In particular, transgender women need to be aware of an increased risk of migraine and should be given advice on effective management in advance of hormone treatment.

9.5   Transgender Hormonal Treatment

Guidelines for management of transgender patients have been produced by the World Professional Association for Transgender Health (WPATH) [11] and the Endocrine Society [1]. It should be noted that these are mostly based on clinical experience rather than evidence-based.

Transgender patients often self-prescribe hormone therapy before referral to a gender clinic [12]. Although this is less common as healthcare professional gains better understanding and experience of prescribing hormones, it remains a problem, particularly among transgender women. In one cross-sectional study in the Netherlands, one in four transgender women self-prescribed treatment, with two-thirds of these obtaining hormones from the Internet [13]. As yet, this is less common in transgender men, in whom the prevalence of self-prescribed hormones was 1 in 17 in the same study. However, this may change as the number of transgender men seeking treatment increases.

Being under the care of a physician is important not just for ensuring the correct dose and monitoring safety but because there is evidence that it can reduce other high-risk behaviours, including smoking cessation and safe needle acquisition [14].

9.5.1   Feminising Hormones for Transgender Women

The goal for feminising hormones is to develop female secondary sex characteristics and suppress male secondary sex characteristics. This is usually achieved using oestrogen together with an androgen blocker. Progestogens are sometimes also used.

Table 9.2 Oestrogen therapy for transgender women

Route	Formulation	Dose (initial–max)
Oral	Oestradiol	2–6 mg/day
Parenteral (subcutaneous or intramuscular)	Oestradiol valerate	5–40 mg every 2 weeks
	Oestradiol cypionate	2.5–10 mg every week
Transdermal	Oestradiol	100–400 µg twice weekly

9.5.1.1 Oestrogen Therapy

Exogenous oestrogen acts through a negative feedback loop to suppress gonadotropin secretion from the pituitary gland, leading to a reduction in androgen production [15]. The aim is to achieve female physiological levels of testosterone (5–55 ng/dL) and oestradiol (100–200 pg/mL). Typical doses and formulations of oestradiol are shown in Table 9.2.

To put these doses into context, the usual maintenance dose of oestrogen for hormone replacement therapy in cisgender women is transdermal 50 µg and oral 2 mg. In addition to migraine, weight gain is a common side effect.

In the past, conjugated equine oestrogens and synthetic ethinylestradiol were used, but the high doses used, particularly of ethinylestradiol (100 µg—three to five times the dose used in current contraceptive formulations), have been associated with increased risk of thrombosis [16, 17]. Further, blood levels are not easy to monitor. Their use has been superseded by 17β oestradiol, which is bioidentical to oestrogen from the human ovary.

Transdermal formulations are recommended as they bypass first-pass metabolism and seem to be associated with better metabolic profiles and are not associated with increased risk of thrombosis [17, 18].

9.5.1.2 Androgen Blockers

Oestrogen alone is insufficient to achieve adequate androgen suppression, so adjunctive anti-androgenic therapy is usually necessary. Spironolactone is the commonest medication used to suppress endogenous testosterone in transgender female patients, which acts by blocking testosterone synthesis and receptor activity. A total daily dose of up to 400 mg daily is usually well tolerated.

Other anti-androgens prescribed include 5-alpha reductase inhibitors such as finasteride, which blocks types 2 and 3 conversion of testosterone to dihydrotestosterone, exerting a much stronger biological activity than does testosterone. Dutasteride is more effective than finasteride as it also blocks the 5-alpha reductase type 1 isozyme, which predominates in the pilosebaceous unit and hence counters male pattern hair loss in favour of a more feminising pattern of hair growth. However, as these drugs do not block testosterone production, they are less effective than spironolactone.

9.5.1.3   Progestogens

Cyproterone acetate is an anti-androgenic progestogen which reduces the effects of androgens by blocking their production in the gonads and also blocking androgen receptors. Depression is a common side effect.

The use of other progestogens is controversial. Medroxyprogesterone acetate (2.5–10 mg daily or 150 mg by intramuscular injection every 3 months) is occasionally prescribed for breast development, but adverse effects include depression, weight gain and adverse lipid changes. Bioidentical micronised progesterone (100–200 mg) daily is an alternative option associated with fewer side effects and a more favourable metabolic profile.

9.5.1.4   Other Drugs

Gonadotrophin-releasing hormone (GnRH) agonists (e.g. goserelin, buserelin) are highly effective at blocking gonadal activity and reducing testosterone levels, but their high cost limits their use.

9.5.1.5   Risks Associated with Feminising Hormones

High doses of oral oestrogen are associated with increased risk of venous thrombosis and cardiovascular and cerebrovascular diseases. These risks may be further increased with co-administration of progestogens. Oral oestrogen has adverse effects on lipids, particularly triglycerides, and may increase blood pressure. This is less likely to occur with transdermal oestrogen [19].

Hyperkalaemia is a potential risk in patients with renal insufficiency using spironolactone co-prescribed with angiotensin-converting enzyme (ACE) inhibitors or angiotensin II receptor blockers (ARBs).

High doses of cyproterone acetate have been associated with increased cardiovascular risk as well as the development of prolactinoma and meningioma [20, 21].

9.5.1.6   Potential Mechanisms of Feminising Hormones on Migraine

Changing plasma levels of oestrogen have been shown in animal models to affect pain thresholds, with higher oestrogen levels associated with lower pain thresholds [22].

Animal studies suggest that high doses of oestrogen increase responses in the trigeminovascular system, a mechanism that may be involved in the headache phase of migraine [23]. Further, oestrogen increases the susceptibility to cortical spreading depression, the pathophysiological mechanism underlying migraine aura [24]. Clinically, this correlates with increased incidence of migraine with aura in high oestrogen states, such as those occurring during pregnancy, with the use of hormone replacement therapy (HRT) and the use of combined hormonal contraception [7]. It may also account for the increased prevalence of aura in transgender women on high-dose oestrogen therapy [8]. For example, high peak plasma oestrogen levels following injection of parenteral oestrogen or high doses of oral oestrogen have the potential to increase risk of aura [7].

In contrast, declining oestrogen towards trough levels can be associated with migraine without aura [7]. While the exact pathophysiology remains largely unknown, oestrogen has potent effects on the serotonin system, increasing serotonergic tone, as well as the opioid system, increasing levels of beta-endorphins [25]. The combination of altered central opioid tonus together with reduced serotonergic tone could potentially increase susceptibility to migraine in states associated with oestrogen withdrawal. In addition, declining perimenstrual oestrogen levels are associated with increased trigeminovascular activity in healthy women [26, 27]. In contrary to what would be expected, such cyclic variations were absent in women with menstrually related migraine [27].

Oestrogen also appears to be involved in regulating sensitisation of trigeminal neurons through mediators such as CGRP, with evidence from animal and human studies that fluctuating oestrogen levels modulate CGRP in both the peripheral and central trigeminovascular systems [28]. Other neuropeptides with purported antinociceptive activity, such as galanin and neuropeptide Y, are expressed at higher levels in high oestrogen states [29]. In these circumstances, oestrogen withdrawal could be associated with a lowered anti-nociceptive environment.

Another potential pathway involves nitric oxide (NO), which can trigger migraine and is also involved with mediating nociceptive transmission [30]. Oestrogen induces NO production via NO synthase activation in the vascular endothelium, resulting in endothelium-dependent vasodilation. In female mice treated with androgens, endothelium-dependent, NO-mediated vasodilator responses are diminished [31], while oestrogen treatment in transgender women has been reported to increase circulating NO levels by 72% [32] and improve endothelium-dependent vasodilation in the forearm resistance circulation [33].

9.5.2 Masculinising Hormones for Transgender Men

The goal for masculinising hormones is to develop male secondary sex characteristics and suppress female secondary sex characteristics. This is usually achieved by using parenteral testosterone. Progestogens, 5-alpha reductase inhibitors or aromatase inhibitors are sometimes also used.

9.5.2.1 Testosterone Therapy

The aim is to achieve testosterone levels in midrange of male norms (350–1000 ng/dL). Typical doses and formulations of testosterone therapy are shown in Table 9.3.

To put these doses into context, the usual maintenance dose of oestrogen for hormone replacement therapy in cisgender women is transdermal 50 µg and oral 2 mg.

Table 9.3 Testosterone therapy for transgender men

Route	Formulation	Dose (initial–max)
Oral	Testosterone undecanoate	160–240 mg/day
Parenteral (subcutaneous or intramuscular)	Testosterone cypionate	50–200 mg/week (or double dose every 2 weeks)
	Testosterone enanthate	50–200 mg/week
Parenteral intramuscular	Testosterone undecanoate[a]	750 mg repeated after 4 weeks then every 10 weeks
Implant (subcutaneous)	Testopel®	75 mg/pellet (6–10 every 3–6 months)
Transdermal	Testosterone gel 1% or cream	12.5–100 mg/day
	Testosterone patch	2–6 mg/day

[a]Off-licence use

Oral testosterone has low bioavailability compared to non-oral formulations and is less effective at suppressing menstruation. Parenteral testosterone cypionate or enanthate can result in cyclic peak and trough effects, particularly when administered at 2-weekly rather than weekly intervals. This does not occur with transdermal testosterone and with intramuscular testosterone undecanoate which both provide stable levels and both result in similar outcomes of masculinisation.

9.5.2.2 Other Drugs

Other hormones used include gonadotropin-releasing hormone (GnRH) agonists and intramuscular depot medroxyprogesterone acetate (150 mg every 3 months). These are given to suppress menstruation, which may be necessary prior to starting testosterone therapy and in the initial stages of treatment.

9.5.2.3 Risks Associated with Masculinising Hormones

Testosterone and androgenic steroids increase the risk of erythrocytosis (secondary polycythaemia), obesity and metabolic syndrome. Headache is a common symptom of polycythaemia, which has been associated with increased risk of migraine aura [34, 35]. These effects may be less likely to occur by more frequent dosing schedules with lower doses of parenteral testosterone to reduce peak levels or by using transdermal routes of delivery.

9.5.2.4 Potential Mechanisms of Masculinising Hormones on Migraine

There is evidence that testosterone reduces chronic pain in transgender men [10]. Preclinical data suggest that testosterone has both anti-nociceptive and anti-inflammatory properties [36, 37]. Additionally, testosterone is known to increase serotonergic tone [38].

The role of testosterone specifically in migraine has been less studied. Mouse models suggest that testosterone suppresses cortical spreading [39], which would potentially be associated with reduced risk of aura. Small studies in humans suggest that treatment with testosterone and its synthetic derivatives may improve migraine in both men and women [40, 41], supporting the finding of reduced risk of migraine in transgender men [10].

9.6 Contraception

Infertility cannot be guaranteed in transgender men or non-binary individuals taking hormone therapy unless they have undergone hysterectomy and/or bilateral oophorectomy. If this group engage in sexual activity that could result in pregnancy, they should be counselled on the need for contraception. Of particular importance is that testosterone is an absolute contraindication for pregnancy due to the risk of masculinisation of a female foetus. The duration of a testosterone washout period for transgender men prior to pregnancy is not known. Progestogen-only methods do not appear to adversely affect masculinising hormone treatment and have the potential benefit of reducing menstruation and risk of migraine [42].

Similarly, transgender women continuing to have vaginal sex with a female partner, who have not undergone orchidectomy or vasectomy, cannot rely on feminising hormones to reduce or block sperm production.

9.7 Management of the Transgender Patient with Migraine

9.7.1 Diagnosis

In transgender patients with headache, it is important that headaches are correctly diagnosed to ensure correct management.

New-onset headache should carefully be evaluated for secondary causes. Evaluation should exclude prolactinoma and meningioma in transgender women and polycythaemia in transgender men. If aura starts for the first time, transient ischaemic attacks should be excluded.

Headaches are not mutually exclusive, and each different headache type should receive a separate diagnosis. The International Headache Society (IHS) has published a classification and diagnostic criteria for migraine and other headache disorders, now in its third edition [43]. While these criteria are important to ensure homogeneity in clinical trials, they are not always practical for use in the clinical setting.

Migraine can more simply be considered as recurrent episodes of disabling headache, lasting 4–72 h associated with nausea and photophobia in an otherwise well person. ID-Migraine™ is a validated diagnostic screening tool based on these key features (Box 9.1) [44, 45].

Box 9.1 'PIN' the Diagnosis of Migraine Without Aura with ID-Migraine™ [44, 45]

*P*hotophobia	Does light bother you when you have a headache?
*I*mpairment	Do you experience headaches that impair your ability to function?
*N*ausea	Do you feel nauseated or sick to your stomach when you have a headache?

In a primary care setting, ID-Migraine™ had a sensitivity of 81% and a specificity of 75% relative to an IHS-based migraine diagnosis assigned by a headache specialist [44]. However, ID-Migraine™ is only a screening tool, and given a false-positive rate of 19%, a more complete evaluation is necessary following a positive result in order to confirm a diagnosis of migraine.

Aura can be more difficult to diagnose as the symptoms are often confused with common premonitory symptoms that precede headache in attacks of both migraine with and without aura [46]. Correct diagnosis of aura is important since aura is a marker of an individual at increased risk of ischaemic stroke [47]. Key aura features are the duration and timing of symptoms in relation to headache (Box 9.2) [48].

Box 9.2 A Simple Screen for Migraine with Aura [48]
Does the patient have visual disturbances that:

Start *before the headache*?
Last *up to 1 h*?
Resolve *before the headache*?

If the answer to all three questions is 'yes', a diagnosis of migraine aura is likely

Visual aura accounts for over 98% of aura symptoms, typically as fortification spectra or a scintillating scotoma starting near the centre of vision and spreading peripherally over 20–30 min.

9.7.2 Managing Migraine

Migraine in transgender men and women is not different from the management of migraine in cisgender patients. National guidelines should be followed accordingly.

9.7.3 Hormone Treatment

In transgender women, stable oestrogen levels are best achieved using non-oral routes of oestradiol administration, which are less likely than oral formulations to trigger migraine. It is important to commence treatment with low doses and increase slowly. Oestrogen injection should be avoided as it can result in significant peak-trough differences [49]. While the high peak oestrogen levels can increase risk of migraine aura [50], falling levels can trigger migraine without aura [51, 52]. This can be mitigated by reducing the injection interval; together with a reduction in dose, transdermal routes are preferred to maintain steady-state dosing [49]. Transdermal routes also have a favourable profile with respect to thrombosis [53]. If aura develops, the oestrogen dose should be reduced where possible, and oral oestrogens, if used, should be switched to transdermal oestrogen.

Of importance is the need to tailor the dose to the individual as there are large inter- and intra-individual variations in serum oestrogen concentrations irrespective of route of administration [49].

In transgender men, the potential benefits of testosterone may not be fully achieved in the absence of full ovarian suppression; fluctuating oestrogen from residual ovarian activity may be sufficient to provoke oestrogen withdrawal migraine even in the absence of menstruation. If this occurs, particularly in the early stages of treatment, additional intramuscular medroxyprogesterone acetate should be considered. Transdermal testosterone is preferred to parenteral testosterone to avoid peak-trough effects.

9.7.4 Reducing Risk

Although there are no specific studies to quantify the risk or the relevant parameters involved, the higher prevalence of aura in transgender women using oestrogen therapy warrants concern. There are no studies of risk associated with transgender treatment; however, three meta-analyses conclude that in cisgender women, migraine with aura is associated with an approximately twofold increased risk of ischaemic stroke (RR 2.08, 95% CI 1.13–3.84) [54–56]. The risk remains increased when analyses control for other major stroke risk factors [57–59]. The addition of oestrogen in doses and routes of delivery that adversely affect coagulation further increases this risk [16, 60].

A particular concern with transgender people is their high use of tobacco [61]. In a case-control study in 22 countries worldwide, current smoking more than doubled the risk of stroke (OR 2.32, 99% CI 1·91–2·81) [62]. Because of the synergism of risks associated with smoking and aura [63], especially if also combined with oestrogen therapy, transgender patients should be counselled about the importance of smoking cessation as well as actively managing other modifiable cardiovascular risk factors.

9.8 Conclusions

The evidence base for the care of transgender men and women with migraine is limited by the paucity of high-quality research, which is needed to inform management guidelines.

The limited data suggest that the prevalence of migraine with and without aura is increased in transgender women treated with oestrogen and is reduced in transgender men treated with testosterone. If migraine does occur, it should be managed according to national guidelines with additional consideration of reducing the impact of hormone therapy. Transdermal oestrogen and testosterone have more favourable metabolic profiles compared to other routes of delivery and should be prescribed in the minimal necessary doses with appropriate monitoring.

There is evidence that aura is associated with increased risk of ischaemic stroke in cisgender women and is further increased by the use of oestrogen and the presence of other risk factors such as smoking. Transgender men and women should be counselled about these potential risks and advised to stop smoking and manage modifiable cardiovascular risk factors.

References

1. Hembree WC, Cohen-Kettenis PT, Gooren L, Hannema SE, Meyer WJ, Murad MH, et al. Endocrine treatment of gender-dysphoric/gender-incongruent persons: an endocrine society clinical practice guideline. J Clin Endocrinol Metab. 2017;102(11):3869–903.
2. American Psychiatric Association. Diagnostic and statistical manual of mental disorders. 5th ed. Arlington, VA: American Psychiatric Association; 2013.
3. Collin L, Reisner SL, Tangpricha V, Goodman M. Prevalence of transgender depends on the "case" definition: a systematic review. J Sex Med. 2016;13(4):613–26.
4. Winter S, Diamond M, Green J, Karasic D, Reed T, Whittle S, et al. Transgender people: health at the margins of society. Lancet. 2016;388(10042):390–400.
5. Gender Identity Development Service. Accessed on 18 Jan 2018. Available from: http://gids.nhs.uk/number-referrals.
6. Vetvik KG, MacGregor EA. Sex differences in the epidemiology, clinical features, and pathophysiology of migraine. Lancet Neurol. 2017;16(1):76–87.
7. MacGregor EA. Oestrogen and attacks of migraine with and without aura. Lancet Neurol. 2004;3(6):354–61.
8. Pringsheim T, Gooren L. Migraine prevalence in male to female transsexuals on hormone therapy. Neurology. 2004;63(3):593–4.
9. Launer LJ, Terwindt GM, Ferrari MD. The prevalence and characteristics of migraine in a population-based cohort: the GEM study. Neurology. 1999;53(3):537–42.
10. Aloisi AM, Bachiocco V, Costantino A, Stefani R, Ceccarelli I, Bertaccini A, et al. Cross-sex hormone administration changes pain in transsexual women and men. Pain. 2007;132(Suppl 1):S60–7.
11. World Professional Association for Transgender Health. Standards of care for the health of transsexual, transgender, and gender nonconforming people. 2011. Accessed on 18 Jan 2018. Available from: https://s3.amazonaws.com/amo_hub_content/Association140/files/Standards%20of%20Care%20V7%20-%202011%20WPATH%20(2)(1).pdf.

12. Sanchez NF, Sanchez JP, Danoff A. Health care utilization, barriers to care, and hormone usage among male-to-female transgender persons in New York City. Am J Public Health. 2009;99(4):713–9.
13. Mepham N, Bouman WP, Arcelus J, Hayter M, Wylie KR. People with gender dysphoria who self-prescribe cross-sex hormones: prevalence, sources, and side effects knowledge. J Sex Med. 2014;11(12):2995–3001.
14. de Haan G, Santos GM, Arayasirikul S, Raymond HF. Non-prescribed hormone use and barriers to care for transgender women in San Francisco. LGBT Health. 2015;2(4):313–23.
15. Dittrich R, Binder H, Cupisti S, Hoffmann I, Beckmann MW, Mueller A. Endocrine treatment of male-to-female transsexuals using gonadotropin-releasing hormone agonist. Exp Clin Endocrinol Diabetes. 2005;113(10):586–92.
16. Asscheman H, Giltay EJ, Megens JA, de Ronde WP, van Trotsenburg MA, Gooren LJ. A long-term follow-up study of mortality in transsexuals receiving treatment with cross-sex hormones. Eur J Endocrinol. 2011;164(4):635–42.
17. Ho JY, Chen MJ, Sheu WH, Yi YC, Tsai AC, Guu HF, et al. Differential effects of oral conjugated equine estrogen and transdermal estrogen on atherosclerotic vascular disease risk markers and endothelial function in healthy postmenopausal women. Hum Reprod. 2006;21(10): 2715–20.
18. Canonico M, Oger E, Plu-Bureau G, Conard J, Meyer G, Levesque H, et al. Hormone therapy and venous thromboembolism among postmenopausal women: impact of the route of estrogen administration and progestogens: the ESTHER study. Circulation. 2007;115(7):840–5.
19. Vehkavaara S, Silveira A, Hakala-Ala-Pietila T, Virkamaki A, Hovatta O, Hamsten A, et al. Effects of oral and transdermal estrogen replacement therapy on markers of coagulation, fibrinolysis, inflammation and serum lipids and lipoproteins in postmenopausal women. Thromb Haemost. 2001;85(4):619–25.
20. Bergoglio MT, Gomez-Balaguer M, Almonacid Folch E, Hurtado Murillo F, Hernandez-Mijares A. Symptomatic meningioma induced by cross-sex hormone treatment in a male-to-female transsexual. Endocrinol Nutr. 2013;60(5):264–7.
21. Goh HH, Li XF, Ratnam SS. Effects of cross-gender steroid hormone treatment on prolactin concentrations in humans. Gynecol Endocrinol. 1992;6(2):113–7.
22. Bradshaw HB, Berkley KJ. The influence of ovariectomy with or without estrogen replacement on responses of rat gracile nucleus neurons to stimulation of hindquarter skin and pelvic viscera. Brain Res. 2003;986(1-2):82–90.
23. Gupta S, Villalon CM, Mehrotra S, de Vries R, Garrelds IM, Saxena PR, et al. Female sex hormones and rat dural vasodilatation to CGRP, periarterial electrical stimulation and capsaicin. Headache. 2007;47(2):225–35.
24. Eikermann-Haerter K, Dilekoz E, Kudo C, Savitz SI, Waeber C, Baum MJ, et al. Genetic and hormonal factors modulate spreading depression and transient hemiparesis in mouse models of familial hemiplegic migraine type 1. J Clin Invest. 2009;119(1):99–109.
25. Sacco S, Ricci S, Degan D, Carolei A. Migraine in women: the role of hormones and their impact on vascular diseases. J Headache Pain. 2012;13(3):177–89.
26. Gazerani P, et al. Pain. 2005;118:155–63.
27. Ibrahimi K, et al. Neurology. 2015;84(2):125–31.
28. Labastida-Ramirez A, Rubio-Beltran E, Villalon CM, MaassenVanDenBrink A. Gender aspects of CGRP in migraine. Cephalalgia. 2017.; 333102417739584.
29. Puri V, Cui L, Liverman CS, Roby KF, Klein RM, Welch KMA, et al. Ovarian steroids regulate neuropeptides in the trigeminal ganglion. Neuropeptides. 2005;39(4):409–17.
30. Goadsby PJ, Holland PR, Martins-Oliveira M, Hoffmann J, Schankin C, Akerman S. Pathophysiology of migraine: a disorder of sensory processing. Physiol Rev. 2017;97(2):553–622.
31. Labruijere S, van Houten EL, de Vries R, Musterd-Bagghoe UM, Garrelds IM, Kramer P, et al. Analysis of the vascular responses in a murine model of polycystic ovary syndrome. J Endocrinol. 2013;218(2):205–13.

32. Valenti S, Fazzuoli L, Giusti M. Circulating nitric oxide levels increase after anti-androgen treatment in male-to-female transsexuals. J Endocrinol Invest. 2003;26(6):522–6.
33. New G, Duffy SJ, Harper RW, Meredith IT. Long-term oestrogen therapy is associated with improved endothelium-dependent vasodilation in the forearm resistance circulation of biological males. Clin Exp Pharmacol Physiol. 2000;27(1-2):25–33.
34. Stanzani Maserati M. Migraine attacks, aura, and polycythemia: a vasculoneural pathogenesis? J Neural Transm (Vienna). 2011;118(4):545–7.
35. Michiels JJ, Berneman Z, Gadisseur A, Lam KH, De Raeve H, Schroyens W. Aspirin-responsive, migraine-like transient cerebral and ocular ischemic attacks and erythromelalgia in JAK2-positive essential thrombocythemia and polycythemia vera. Acta Haematol. 2015;133(1):56–63.
36. Cairns BE, Gazerani P. Sex-related differences in pain. Maturitas. 2009;63(4):292–6.
37. Gupta S, McCarson KE, Welch KM, Berman NE. Mechanisms of pain modulation by sex hormones in migraine. Headache. 2011;51(6):905–22.
38. Fink G, Sumner B, Rosie R, Wilson H, McQueen J. Androgen actions on central serotonin neurotransmission: relevance for mood, mental state and memory. Behav Brain Res. 1999;105(1):53–68.
39. Eikermann-Haerter K, Baum MJ, Ferrari MD, van den Maagdenberg AM, Moskowitz MA, Ayata C. Androgenic suppression of spreading depression in familial hemiplegic migraine type 1 mutant mice. Ann Neurol. 2009;66(4):564–8.
40. Lichten EM, Bennett RS, Whitty AJ, Daoud Y. Efficacy of danazol in the control of hormonal migraine. J Reprod Med. 1991;36(6):419–24.
41. Glaser R, Dimitrakakis C, Trimble N, Martin V. Testosterone pellet implants and migraine headaches: a pilot study. Maturitas. 2012;71(4):385–8.
42. Merki-Feld GS, Imthurn B, Langner R, Seifert B, Gantenbein AR. Positive effects of the progestin desogestrel 75 mg on migraine frequency and use of acute medication are sustained over a treatment period of 180 days. J Headache Pain. 2015;16:522.
43. Headache Classification Committee of the International Headache Society (IHS). The International Classification of Headache Disorders, 3rd edition. Cephalalgia. 2018;38(1):1–211.
44. Lipton RB, Dodick D, Sadovsky R, Kolodner K, Endicott J, Hettiarachchi J, et al. A self-administered screener for migraine in primary care: the ID Migraine validation study. Neurology. 2003;61(3):375–82.
45. Dodick DW. Pearls: headache. Semin Neurol. 2010;30(1):74–81.
46. Blau JN. Migraine: theories of pathogenesis. Lancet. 1992;339(8803):1202–7.
47. Kurth T, Chabriat H, Bousser MG. Migraine and stroke: a complex association with clinical implications. Lancet Neurol. 2012;11(1):92–100.
48. Gervil M, Ulrich V, Olesen J, Russell M. Screening for migraine in the general population: validation of a simple questionnaire. Cephalalgia. 1998;18:342–8.
49. Kuhl H. Pharmacokinetics of oestrogen and progestogens. Maturitas. 1990;12:171–97.
50. MacGregor A. Estrogen replacement and migraine aura. Headache. 1999;39:674–8.
51. Somerville BW. The role of estradiol withdrawal in the etiology of menstrual migraine. Neurology. 1972;22(4):355–65.
52. Lichten EM, Lichten JB, Whitty A, Pieper D. The confirmation of a biochemical marker for women's hormonal migraine: the depo-estradiol challenge test. Headache. 1996;36(6):367–71.
53. van Kesteren PJ, Asscheman H, Megens JA, Gooren LJ. Mortality and morbidity in transsexual subjects treated with cross-sex hormones. Clin Endocrinol (Oxf). 1997;47(3):337–42.
54. Schurks M, Rist PM, Bigal ME, Buring JE, Lipton RB, Kurth T. Migraine and cardiovascular disease: systematic review and meta-analysis. BMJ. 2009;339:b3914.
55. Spector JT, Kahn SR, Jones MR, Jayakumar M, Dalal D, Nazarian S. Migraine headache and ischemic stroke risk: an updated meta-analysis. Am J Med. 2010;123(7):612–24.
56. Etminan M, Takkouche B, Isorna FC, Samii A. Risk of ischaemic stroke in people with migraine: systematic review and meta-analysis of observational studies. BMJ. 2005;330(7482):63–5.

57. Kurth T, Schurks M, Logroscino G, Gaziano JM, Buring JE. Migraine, vascular risk, and car-diovascular events in women: prospective cohort study. BMJ. 2008;337:a636.
58. Bigal ME, Kurth T, Santanello N, Buse D, Golden W, Robbins M, et al. Migraine and cardio-vascular disease: a population-based study. Neurology. 2010;74(8):628–35.
59. Li L, Schulz UG, Kuker W, Rothwell PM, Oxford Vascular S. Age-specific associa-tion of migraine with cryptogenic TIA and stroke: population-based study. Neurology. 2015;85(17):1444–51.
60. Rossouw JE, Anderson GL, Prentice RL, LaCroix AZ, Kooperberg C, Stefanick ML, et al. Risks and benefits of estrogen plus progestin in healthy postmenopausal women: principal results From the Women's Health Initiative randomized controlled trial. JAMA. 2002;288(3):321–33.
61. Clarke MP, Coughlin JR. Prevalence of smoking among the lesbian, gay, bisexual, transsexual, transgender and queer (LGBTTQ) subpopulations in Toronto--the Toronto Rainbow Tobacco Survey (TRTS). Can J Public Health. 2012;103(2):132–6.
62. O'Donnell MJ, Xavier D, Liu L, Zhang H, Chin SL, Rao-Melacini P, et al. Risk factors for ischaemic and intracerebral haemorrhagic stroke in 22 countries (the INTERSTROKE study): a case-control study. Lancet. 2010;376(9735):112–23.
63. Scher AI, Terwindt GM, Picavet HS, Verschuren WM, Ferrari MD, Launer LJ. Cardiovascular risk factors and migraine: the GEM population-based study. Neurology. 2005;64(4):614–20.